Intensive Care Medicine

MCQs

Multiple Choice Questions with Explanatory Answers

Editor:

Steve Benington MBChB MRCP FRCA EDIC FFICM

Authors:

Shoneen Abbas MBChB MRCP FFICM

Ruth Herod MBChB FRCA FFICM

Daniel Horner BA MBBS MD MRCP(UK) FCEM FFICM

tfm Publishing Limited, Castle Hill Barns, Harley, Shrewsbury, SY5 6LX, UK
Tel: +44 (0)1952 510061; Fax: +44 (0)1952 510192
E-mail: info@tfmpublishing.com
Web site: www.tfmpublishing.com

Editing, design & typesetting: Nikki Bramhill BSc Hons Dip Law
First edition: © 2015
Front cover image: © 2015 Sudok1/Dreamstime.com LLC
Paperback   ISBN: 978-1-910079-07-2
E-book editions: 2015
ePub   ISBN: 978-1-910079-08-9
Mobi   ISBN: 978-1-910079-09-6
Web pdf   ISBN: 978-1-910079-10-2

Printed by Gutenberg Press Ltd., Gudja Road, Tarxien, PLA 19, Malta

Contents

Preface

This book contains three 90-question multiple choice papers designed to test the candidate's knowledge of intensive care medicine (ICM) and their ability to apply it. Each paper begins with 60 multiple true false (MTF) questions consisting of a stem and five statements, each requiring a true or false answer. These are followed by 30 single best answer (SBA) questions where a clinical vignette is presented with five possible solutions. The candidate should select the one that best addresses the problem, mirroring clinical practice where a case usually has several possible approaches.

Topics have been chosen to cover the breadth of knowledge required of the modern intensivist, including resuscitation, diagnosis, disease management, organ support, applied anatomy, end-of-life care and applied basic sciences. There is a strong focus on the evidence base underpinning the specialty, making this book particularly useful for physicians and others approaching professional examinations in ICM and related acute medical and surgical specialties. There is no 'pass mark', although a score of less than four out of five in an MTF question or an incorrect response to an SBA question should help the candidate identify areas where they would benefit from further reading. Each question is accompanied by a detailed and fully referenced answer; the majority of references are freely accessible online or through institutional subscriptions.

The authors are all senior trainees or consultants practising intensive care medicine in the UK with firsthand experience of passing professional examinations. In addition, they have extensive training and experience in acute medicine, anaesthesia and emergency medicine, respectively, and have drawn on their experience to devise questions that reflect these specialties and their interface with intensive care medicine. The authors hope that this book will be a useful resource not only for those approaching examinations but for anyone wishing to keep up-to-date in this fast-changing specialty.

Steve Benington MBChB MRCP FRCA EDIC FFICM
Shoneen Abbas MBChB MRCP FFICM
Ruth Herod MBChB FRCA FFICM
Daniel Horner BA MBBS MD MRCP(UK) FCEM FFICM

Acknowledgements

The Editor would like to thank Dr Ola Abbas and Dr Fiona Wallace for their invaluable help proofreading the manuscript. Also, thanks to Dr John Macdonald, Dr Hakeem Yousuff, Dr Richard Ramsaran and Dr Andrew Martin for their comments while testing the questions.

Abbreviations

The following are the most commonly used abbreviations throughout the book:

AAGBI	Association of Anaesthetists of Great Britain and Ireland
ABG	Arterial blood gas
ACS	Abdominal compartment syndrome
ACTH	Adrenocorticotropic hormone
AF	Atrial fibrillation
AFE	Amniotic fluid embolism
AFLP	Acute fatty liver of pregnancy
AIS	Abbreviated Injury Scale
AKI	Acute kidney injury
ALF	Acute liver failure
ALI	Acute lung injury
ALS	Advanced Life Support
AP	Acute pancreatitis
APACHE	Acute Physiology and Chronic Health Evaluation
APLS	Advanced Paediatric Life Support
APRV	Airway pressure release ventilation
aPTT	Activated partial thromboplastin time
ARDS	Acute respiratory distress syndrome
ARR	Absolute risk reduction
ASIA	American Spinal Injury Association
AT	Anaerobic threshold
ATLS	Advanced Trauma Life Support
ATN	Acute tubular necrosis
BE	Base excess
BMI	Body mass index
BNP	B-natriuretic peptide
BP	Blood pressure
BTS	British Thoracic Society
CAM-ICU	Confusion Assessment Method for the Intensive Care Unit
cAMP	Cyclic adenosine monophosphate

CAP	Community-acquired pneumonia
CDI	*Clostridium difficile* infection
cGMP	Cyclic guanosine monophosphate
CIN	Contrast-induced nephropathy
CK	Creatine kinase
CKD	Chronic kidney disease
Cl⁻	Chloride
CMAP	Compound muscle action potential
CMV	*Cytomegalovirus*
COPD	Chronic obstructive pulmonary disease
CPAP	Continuous positive airway pressure
CPET	Cardiopulmonary exercise testing
CPIS	Clinical Pulmonary Infection Score
CPK	Creatinine phosphokinase
CPP	Cerebral perfusion pressure
CPR	Cardiopulmonary resuscitation
CRP	C-reactive protein
CRRT	Continuous renal replacement therapy
CSF	Cerebrospinal fluid
CT	Computed tomography
CTPA	Computed tomography pulmonary angiogram
CVC	Central venous catheter
CVP	Central venous pressure
CXR	Chest X-ray
DBD	Donation after brainstem death
DCD	Donation after cardiac death
DDAVP	Desmopressin
DI	Diabetes insipidus
DIC	Disseminated intravascular coagulation
DKA	Diabetic ketoacidosis
DVT	Deep vein thrombosis
ECG	Electrocardiogram
ECMO	Extracorporeal membrane oxygenation
EEG	Electroencephalography
EMG	Electromyography
ESR	Erythrocyte sedimentation rate
ETCO$_2$	End-tidal carbon dioxide
EVD	External ventricular drain
FFP	Fresh frozen plasma
FRC	Functional residual capacity
HR	Heart rate

GBS	Guillain-Barré syndrome
GCS	Glasgow Coma Scale
GFR	Glomerular filtration rate
GMC	General Medical Council
GTN	Glyceryl trinitrate
HAS	Human albumin solution
HCM	Hypertrophic cardiomyopathy
HFOV	High-frequency oscillatory ventilation
HME	Heat and moisture exchangers
HRS	Hepatorenal syndrome
IABP	Intra-aortic balloon pump
IAH	Intra-abdominal hypertension
IAP	Intra-abdominal pressure
ICP	Intracranial pressure
ICU	Intensive care unit
ICUAW	Intensive care unit-acquired weakness
ILCOR	International Liaison Committee on Resuscitation
INR	International Normalised Ratio
ISS	Injury Severity Score
K^+	Potassium
KDIGO	The Kidney Disease: Improving Global Outcomes
LDH	Lactate dehydrogenase
LMA	Laryngeal mask airway
LMWH	Low-molecular-weight heparin
LP	Lumbar puncture
LQTS	Long QT syndrome
LVOT	Left ventricular outflow tract
MAP	Mean arterial pressure
MDR	Multidrug resistance
MELD	Modified End-stage Liver Disease
MEN	Multiple endocrine neoplasia
MEOWS	Modified Early Obstetric Warning Score
MET	Metabolic equivalent
MG	Myasthenia gravis
Mg^{2+}	Magnesium
MH	Malignant hyperthermia
MHRA	Medicines and Healthcare Products Regulatory Agency
MI	Myocardial infarction
MODS	Multiple Organ Dysfunction Score
MPAP	Mean pulmonary artery pressure
MPM	Mortality Prediction Model

MRC	Medical Research Council
MRI	Magnetic resonance imaging
MRSA	Methicillin-resistant *Staphylococcus aureus*
NICE	The National Institute for Health and Care Excellence
NIV	Non-invasive ventilation
Na$^+$	Sodium
NAC	N-acetyl cysteine
NF	Necrotizing fasciitis
NHSBT	National Health Service Blood and Transplant
NICE	National Institute for Health and Care Excellence
NMS	Neuroleptic malignant syndrome
NNT	Number needed to treat
NPV	Negative predictive value
NSAID	Non-steroidal anti-inflammatory drug
PAC	Pulmonary artery catheter
PAOP	Pulmonary artery occlusion pressure
PCI	Primary coronary intervention
PCR	Polymerase chain reaction
PCV	Pressure-controlled ventilation
PCWP	Pulmonary capillary wedge pressure
PE	Pulmonary embolism
PEEP	Positive end-expiratory pressure
PEFR	Peak expiratory flow rate
P:F ratio	Ratio of partial pressure of arterial oxygen to fraction of inspired oxygen
PLR	Passive leg raising
PN	Parenteral nutrition
POSSUM	Physiological and Operative Severity Score for the enUmeration of Mortality and Morbidity
PPI	Proton pump inhibitor
Pplat	Plateau pressure
PPV	Positive predictive value
PRIS	Propofol infusion syndrome
PT	Prothrombin time
PTHrP	Parathyroid hormone-related protein
QALY	Quality-adjusted life-year
RASS	Richmond Agitation Severity Scale
RCT	Randomised controlled trial
rFVIIa	Recombinant Factor VIIa
RIFLE	Risk, Injury, Failure, Loss, End-stage renal disease
ROC	Receiver operator characteristic

ROSC	Return of spontaneous circulation
ROSIER	Recognition of Stroke in the Emergency Room
RR	Respiratory rate
RSBI	Rapid Shallow Breathing Index
RTS	Revised Trauma Score
SAH	Subarachnoid haemorrhage
SAPS	Simplified Acute Physiology Score
$ScvO_2$	Central venous oxygen saturation
SDD	Selective digestive tract decontamination
SIADH	Syndrome of inappropriate antidiuretic hormone secretion
SID	Strong ion difference
SLE	Systemic lupus erythematosus
SNAP	Sensory (or mixed) nerve action potential
SOFA	Sequential Organ Failure Assessment
STEMI	ST elevation myocardial infarction
SVC	Superior vena cava
SVRI	Systemic vascular resistance index
TBI	Traumatic brain injury
TBSA	Total body surface area
TEG	Thromboelastography
TIA	Transient ischaemic attack
TIPSS	Transjugular intrahepatic portosystemic shunting
TISS	Therapeutic Intervention Scoring System
TLS	Tumour lysis syndrome
TRISS	Trauma Injury Severity Score
TSS	Toxic shock syndrome
TTP	Thrombotic thrombocytopaenia purpura
VAD	Ventricular assist device
VAP	Ventilator-associated pneumonia
VATS	Video-assisted thoracoscopic surgery
VCV	Volume-controlled ventilation
VF	Ventricular fibrillation
VT	Ventricular tachycardia
Vt	Tidal volume
VTE	Venous thromboembolism
vWF	von Willebrand Factor
WCC	White cell count
WFNS	World Federation of Neurosurgeons
WPW	Wolff-Parkinson-White
WSACS	World Society of the Abdominal Compartment Syndrome

Converting units of measurement

Laboratory results presented in the questions are given in standard UK units. The following conversion factors may be useful to readers from other areas:

$1\mu mol/L = 0.0113mg/dL$ (e.g. serum bilirubin, creatinine)

$1kPa = 7.5mmHg$ (e.g. PaO_2)

Topic index

Multiple True False (MTF) questions — select true or false for each of the five stems.

1 Guillain-Barré syndrome (GBS):

a. Affects more females than males.
b. Is a disease of the middle-aged.
c. When secondary to a respiratory illness, the majority of cases present within a month.
d. The presence of cranial nerve signs effectively rules out the diagnosis.
e. The most common associated pathogen is *Clostridium perfringens*.

2 In the trauma patient with massive haemorrhage, the following statements are correct:

a. An initial target systolic blood pressure of 80-90mmHg is recommended for the patient without brain injury.
b. Desmopressin at a dose of 0.3µg/kg is recommended in the bleeding patient taking platelet-inhibiting drugs.
c. Recombinant factor VIIa (rFVIIa) can be considered as a rescue measure provided the platelet count is greater than 30 x 10⁹/L.
d. Pre-injury warfarin use doubles the odds of death for trauma patients with blunt head injury.
e. Antifibrinolytic drugs recommended for use in the bleeding major trauma patient include tranexamic acid, aprotinin and aminocaproic acid.

3 The following drugs undergo non-organ metabolism:

a. Esmolol.
b. Atracurium.
c. Inhaled nitric oxide.
d. Propofol.
e. Adrenaline.

4 Which of the following features of an asthma attack are classified as 'life-threatening' in the 2011 BTS asthma guideline?

a. Inability to complete sentences in one breath.
b. PaO_2 of >8kPa.
c. Silent chest.
d. $PaCO_2$ >6kPa.
e. Peak expiratory flow rate (PEFR) <50% of predicted.

5 With regard to bleeding and coagulopathy in the critically ill patient:

a. If a platelet transfusion is indicated, 1 unit will raise the count by approximately 20×10^9/L.
b. The principal constituents of cryoprecipitate include Factors VIII, XIII, vWF, fibronectin and fibrinogen.
c. A suggested dose of fresh frozen plasma in the bleeding trauma patient with coagulopathy is 30ml/kg.
d. Desmopressin at a dose of 0.3µg/kg is a useful treatment in patients with coagulopathy related to uraemia, cirrhosis and aspirin use.
e. At temperatures of 33-35°C, altered enzyme kinetics equate to a 33% reduction in normal clotting factors.

6   Regarding drug-receptor interactions:

a. An antagonist has receptor affinity and intrinsic activity.
b. Increasing the dose of a partial agonist can elicit a maximal effect.
c. β-receptor blockers are reversible antagonists.
d. Flumazenil is an inverse agonist.
e. Phenoxybenzamine is an irreversible antagonist at α-adrenoceptors.

7   Regarding the hepatorenal syndrome (HRS):

a. It is commonly over-diagnosed in patients with cirrhotic liver disease.
b. HRS Type 1 has the poorest outcome.
c. Kidneys from patients with HRS are suitable for transplantation.
d. The condition is associated with splanchnic vasodilatation.
e. Terlipressin must be given by infusion.

8   With regard to a patient with a neuromuscular disorder on the critical care unit:

a. Potassium-sparing diuretics should be avoided in patients with hypokalaemic periodic paralysis.
b. Suxamethonium use should be avoided in patients with myasthenia gravis.
c. Patients with motor neurone disease typically require double the standard dose of suxamethonium to provide optimum intubating conditions.
d. Local anaesthesia can exacerbate symptoms of multiple sclerosis.
e. In Guillain-Barré syndrome, non-depolarising neuromuscular blocking drugs may be used, but should be significantly dose-reduced.

9 Regarding parenteral nutrition in the critically ill patient:

a. A patient with enteral feeds running at 40ml/hr with 4-hourly aspirates of >200ml is deemed to be failing enteral nutrition.
b. Daily caloric intake should be 100-130% of the patient's calculated daily energy expenditure.
c. Parenteral nutrition can be administered peripherally.
d. Approximately 1g/kg/day of nitrogen is required.
e. Copper, zinc and selenium (trace elements) are present in commercially produced parenteral nutrition solutions.

10 A 67-year-old male has a diagnosis of myasthenia gravis (MG). Which of the following medications should be avoided to reduce the risk of exacerbation?

a. Gentamicin.
b. Paracetamol.
c. Trimethoprim.
d. Ciprofloxacin.
e. Aspirin.

11 The following statements are true regarding the management of acute severe asthma:

a. PEFR <33% is a criterion diagnosis.
b. Aminophylline should be given as a first-line intravenous bronchodilator.
c. The use of IV magnesium sulphate to reduce mortality is supported by level I evidence.
d. Ketamine 5mg/kg is the preferred induction agent if rapid sequence intubation is required.
e. A restrictive fluid regime should be used in patients at risk of intubation.

12 Regarding the role of selective digestive tract decontamination (SDD) on the ICU:

a. Eight potentially pathogenic micro-organisms are responsible for the majority of infections in critical care.
b. SDD is 'selective' because it is anaerobe-sparing.
c. Primary endogenous pathogens are targeted by intravenous antibiotics for the first 4 days.
d. After 10 days potentially pathogenic micro-organisms have been eradicated and all antibiotics are stopped.
e. There is level I evidence that SDD increases the prevalence of antibiotic resistance.

13 A 59-year-old male is admitted with a gradual onset of peripheral oedema and frothy urine. He is subsequently diagnosed with nephrotic syndrome. The condition is associated with:

a. Hypercalcaemia.
b. Venous thrombosis.
c. Hyperlipidaemia.
d. Risk of myocardial infarction.
e. Hypervolaemia.

14 The following have been demonstrated to be useful prognostic variables in moderate to severe traumatic brain injury:

a. Age.
b. Pupillary reaction.
c. Sensory neurological deficit.
d. The presence of non-evacuated haematoma on CT brain scan.
e. Serum glucose.

15 Regarding the use of ventricular assist devices (VADs) for the management of acute and chronic heart failure:

a.   Ventricular assist devices can be used for a maximum of 3-4 weeks.
b.   A short-term left ventricular assist device takes blood from the right atrium and injects it into the main pulmonary artery.
c.   Most modern ventricular assist devices produce a pulsatile flow.
d.   The insertion of an LVAD worsens aortic regurgitation.
e.   All patients with VADs must be anticoagulated.

16 Regarding diagnostic lumbar puncture (LP):

a.   Meningitis is a relatively rare complication of LP.
b.   Suspected bacteraemia is a contraindication to LP.
c.   Aspirin should be stopped for at least 24 hours prior to LP.
d.   LP is contraindicated in patients with a suspected spinal epidural abscess.
e.   It is recommended that LP is not performed in patients with platelet counts of <100 x 10^9.

17 With regard to intracranial pressure (ICP) monitoring:

a.   Ocular nerve sheath diameter >6mm measured with ultrasound reliably predicts raised intracranial pressure of >20mmHg.
b.   ICP monitoring through an external ventricular drain allows therapeutic intervention.
c.   On a standard intracranial pressure waveform, P3 represents cerebral compliance.
d.   Cerebral hypoxia results in hypoxic vasoconstriction and reduced cerebral blood flow, thus causing a temporary reduction in ICP.
e.   Lundberg Type A waves are always pathological.

18 Regarding the mechanics of positive pressure ventilation:

a.   Setting an extrinsic positive end-expiratory pressure (PEEP) less than intrinsic PEEP will reduce elastic work of the respiratory system.
b.   One risk of applying PEEP is a reduction in oxygen delivery (DO_2).
c.   A decelerating flow pattern is seen in volume-controlled ventilation.
d.   The difference between peak and plateau pressures is greater with volume-controlled ventilation than pressure-controlled ventilation.
e.   Dynamic compliance equals the tidal volume divided by (peak pressure minus total positive end-expiratory pressure).

19 The following are examples of severity scoring systems in the intensive care unit:

a.   Acute Physiology and Chronic Health Evaluation III (APACHE III).
b.   CT Calcium Score.
c.   Sequential Organ Failure Assessment (SOFA).
d.   Mortality Prediction Model (MPM).
e.   Glasgow-Blatchford Score.

20 The following are examples of superiority randomised controlled trials (RCTs) relevant to critical care, whose results support the proposed null hypothesis:

a.   ProCESS.
b.   PROSEVA.
c.   TTM.
d.   VASST.
e.   OSCAR.

21 Regarding plasma exchange:

a. It is a highly effective treatment for thrombotic thrombocytopaenic purpura.
b. The most commonly used replacement fluid is 4.5% albumin in physiological saline.
c. Therapeutic plasma exchange requires central venous access.
d. Paraesthesia is a common complication.
e. Thrombosis is a common complication.

22 In patients with, or at risk of, acute kidney injury (AKI), international consensus guidelines suggest the following:

a. In critically ill patients, insulin therapy should target a plasma glucose of about 6-8mmol/L.
b. Administration of colloid boluses to expand intravascular volume.
c. Parenteral nutrition should be used in preference to the enteral route in patients with AKI.
d. N-acetyl cysteine (NAC) should not be used for the prevention of post-surgical AKI.
e. Low-dose dopamine has a role in the treatment of established AKI.

23 With regard to the Medical Research Council-funded CRASH trials:

a. The CRASH 1 trial examined the role of steroids in traumatic brain injury (TBI).
b. The CRASH 2 trial assessed the role of tranexamic acid in traumatic brain injury (TBI) within a pilot sample.
c. The CRASH 3 trial is designed to assess the effectiveness of tranexamic acid in TBI within a multicentre cohort.

d.   The number needed to treat (NNT) in Crash 2 to save one life was >50.
e.   There is now level I evidence to support the role of steroids in TBI.

24 Regarding diabetic ketoacidosis (DKA):

a.   DKA can be diagnosed if a known diabetic patient presents with hyperglycaemia (plasma glucose >10mmol/L) and a serum bicarbonate of <15mmol/L.
b.   A high serum ketone level indicates more severe disease.
c.   DKA should be treated with a fixed rate insulin infusion.
d.   When managing a patient with DKA, their usual insulin regime should be stopped but oral antidiabetic medication should be continued.
e.   DKA is deemed to have resolved when urinary ketones are no longer detectable.

25 The following apply to levosimendan:

a.   It impairs diastolic relaxation.
b.   It is a sodium channel sensitiser.
c.   It increases myocardial oxygen consumption.
d.   It can be used with β-blockers.
e.   No loading dose is required due to the very short half-life.

26 With regard to thrombotic thrombocytopaenia purpura (TTP):

a.   Platelet transfusion is recommended to maintain a platelet count of >10 x 10^9/L.

b.   The principal abnormality occurs due to the production of an abnormal vWF cleaving protein.
c.   The diagnostic pentad includes microangiopathic haemolytic anaemia.
d.   The diagnostic pentad includes proven or suspected arterial or venous thrombosis.
e.   Administration of solvent/detergent-treated fresh frozen plasma is a useful treatment option.

27 Anatomical landmarks and anatomy in relation to therapeutic practical procedures are as follows:

a.   Needle decompression of a tension pneumothorax is best performed by inserting a needle immediately below the second rib in the mid-axillary line.
b.   A chest drain should be inserted in the 5th intercostal space, just anterior to the mid-axillary line.
c.   Abdominal paracentesis can safely be performed 1cm below the umbilicus.
d.   A central venous catheter inserted into the femoral vein will lie medial to the femoral nerve and lateral to the femoral artery.
e.   Needle insertion for landmark-guided pericardiocentesis is immediately below and to the right of the xiphisternum, between the xiphisternum and the right costal margin.

28 A 67-year-old male has been mechanically ventilated for 2 weeks on the ICU. He has had multiple courses of antibiotics for chest sepsis. He develops profuse diarrhoea over 2 days. A diagnosis of *Clostridium difficile* infection is considered. Regarding this organism:

a.   Around 20% of all cases of antibiotic-associated diarrhoea are due to *Clostridium difficile*.

b. β-lactam antibiotics are least commonly associated with *Clostridium difficile* infection.
c. The onset of diarrhoea may not occur until several weeks after the termination of antibiotic therapy.
d. Stool culture has a high specificity but low sensitivity for diagnosis.
e. Asymptomatic carriage of *C. difficile* among hospitalised patients is low.

29 Regarding the acute management of a subarachnoid haemorrhage:

a. The peak incidence of vasospasm occurs at day 4.
b. Use of intravenous magnesium to reduce the incidence of vasospasm is supported by the MASH (Magnesium for Aneurysmal Subarachnoid Haemorrhage) trials.
c. Hypervolaemia, hypertension and haemodilution therapy reduces the incidence of vasospasm.
d. Mean arterial pressure (MAP) targets should be set to >90mmHg following protection of the aneurysm.
e. Clipping and coiling are equally effective treatment options in terms of neurological outcome.

30 Regarding the pre-operative assessment of exercise capacity:

a. 1 metabolic equivalent (MET) is roughly equivalent to climbing one flight of stairs.
b. The anaerobic threshold (AT) is the point at which oxygen supply exceeds demand.
c. Patients with an AT of >15ml/min O_2 have a high relative risk of cardiopulmonary morbidity following major non-cardiac surgery.
d. Cardiopulmonary exercise testing is relatively contraindicated in the presence of severe aortic stenosis.
e. Oxygen consumption = cardiac output x (arterial-mixed venous oxygen content).

31 A patient on the cardiothoracic intensive care unit has an intra-aortic balloon pump (IABP) *in situ*. Which of the following apply with regard to the IABP?

a. An IABP is contraindicated in aortic stenosis.
b. The IABP can be inserted via the femoral route.
c. The balloon inflates during systole.
d. Heliox is used to inflate the balloon.
e. An IABP improves cerebral and coronary perfusion.

32 In a patient with acute severe tricyclic antidepressant poisoning:

a. A dominant R-wave >3mm is often seen in lead aVR.
b. QRS prolongation is a useful prognostic feature and should be routinely measured.
c. First-line treatment for acute dysrhythmia should include a 2-4g bolus of magnesium sulphate.
d. Intralipid® can be used as a rescue measure.
e. The pH should be normalised by intubation and hyperventilation.

33 Regarding the physiology of the donor heart following cardiac transplantation:

a. β-adrenergic blockers will have no effect on the heart rate.
b. The Valsalva manoeurvre will have no effect on heart rate.
c. Glyceryl trinitrate (GTN) will cause coronary vasodilatation.
d. The post-cardiac transplant patient can suffer anginal pain.
e. The heart rate will not increase during exercise unless a pacemaker is fitted.

34 A 79-year-old female suffers a cardiopulmonary arrest on the medical ward. She is in ventricular fibrillation. The team is struggling with venous access. Full cardiopulmonary resuscitation (CPR) is in progress. The patient is intubated. According to the Advanced Life Support (ALS) 2010 resuscitation guidelines, the following are recommended:

a. A precordial thump.
b. Administration of emergency drugs via the endotracheal tube.
c. Intraosseous access as a route of drug delivery.
d. Administration of 1mg adrenaline after the third DC shock.
e. Amiodarone after the fourth DC shock.

35 The following are recognised complications of therapeutic hypothermia:

a. Pneumonia.
b. Coagulopathy.
c. Hypoglycaemia.
d. Sepsis.
e. Renal failure.

36 Regarding the pathophysiology, management and treatment of necrotising fasciitis:

a. Mortality is directly proportional to time to intervention.
b. The most common type of necrotising fasciitis is caused by Group A *Streptococcus* (*Streptococcus pyogenes*).
c. Skin changes are a common early presentation of necrotising fasciitis.
d. Surgical debridement must be performed as antibiotics are unable to penetrate the infected necrotic tissue.
e. Clindamycin is first-line monotherapy.

37 In a patient with suspected rhabdomyolysis:

a. The absence of myoglobinuria excludes the diagnosis.
b. Administration of sodium bicarbonate and mannitol are the mainstays of treatment.
c. Alkalinisation of the urine aims to increase the solubility of the Tamm-Horsfall protein-myoglobin complex.
d. Bicarbonate should be titrated to a urinary pH >9.
e. Hypercalcaemia is frequently seen in the early stages.

38 Regarding the prevention and grading of pressure ulcers in the critically ill:

a. Pressure, shear and friction are all required for a pressure ulcer to develop.
b. The Waterlow score is used to grade pressure ulcers.
c. All grade I pressure ulcers have intact skin.
d. The APACHE II score correlates well with the occurrence of pressure ulcers.
e. Critically ill patients should be turned every 2-3 hours to prevent the development of pressure ulcers, if their clinical condition allows.

39 A patient presents with a paracetamol overdose. The following factors would increase the chances of severe hepatotoxicity:

a. High body mass index.
b. Regular consumption of ethanol in excess of recommended amounts.
c. Use of hepatic enzyme inhibitors.
d. Malnourishment.
e. St John's Wort.

40 With respect to the tumour lysis syndrome (TLS):

a. High-dose intravenous steroid therapy is a reasonable initial treatment option.
b. TLS is most commonly associated with squamous cell and neuroendocrine tumours.
c. Clinical TLS can be diagnosed in a patient with seizures and the presence of appropriate laboratory findings.
d. An increase in serum calcium and potassium levels by >25% is the hallmark feature of laboratory TLS.
e. Allopurinol is the treatment of choice for preventing acute kidney injury in TLS.

41 The following are diagnostic features of submassive pulmonary embolism (PE):

a. Dilated right ventricle on echocardiography.
b. Systolic blood pressure <90mmHg.
c. Elevated troponin.
d. B-natriuretic peptide (BNP) level of <10pg/ml.
e. SpO_2 <94% on room air.

42 Regarding the diagnosis of brainstem death:

a. Fixed and dilated pupils must be present.
b. The absence of corneal reflex indicates no function in the midbrain region.
c. The visual evoked responses must be demonstrated to be absent.
d. Motor response to a sternal rub excludes the diagnosis.
e. A cough reflex response to bronchial stimulation by a suction catheter placed down the trachea to the carina excludes the diagnosis.

43 The following factors cause inaccuracy in pulse oximetry:

a. Methaemoglobinaemia.
b. Carbon monoxide poisoning.
c. Vasopressors.
d. Acrylic nails.
e. Hyperbilirubinaemia.

44 The following are considered useful management options in the treatment of thrombotic thrombocytopaenia purpura (TTP):

a. Intravenous immunoglobulin.
b. Steroid therapy.
c. Platelet transfusion.
d. Monoclonal antibody infusion.
e. Fresh frozen plasma.

45 Regarding the ethical and legal aspects of organ donation after cardiac death and after brainstem death in the UK:

a. Once the decision for organ donation in a brainstem dead patient has been made, management should move from a 'patient-focused approach' to an 'organ management approach'.
b. Regarding donation after cardiac death, it is ethically acceptable to delay the process of withdrawal in the donor until the donor process is in place.
c. Verbal expression of a wish to donate organs expressed before death is a valid form of consent for organ retrieval after death.

d.   The family does not have legal authority to refuse organ donation if the dead patient previously consented to this.
e.   Patients must be at least 16 years of age to register on the Organ Donor Register.

46 **The following are appropriate for the resuscitation of the average 4-year-old child:**

a.   Size 5 uncuffed endotracheal tube.
b.   In the case of witnessed ventricular fibrillation, synchronised defibrillation at 64 Joules.
c.   In a cardiac arrest, 160µg adrenaline, IO or IV.
d.   Lorazepam 1.6mg/kg IV for the emergency treatment of convulsions.
e.   Atropine 640µg for the emergency treatment of bradycardia suspected to be due to vagal overactivity.

47 **In the diagnosis and management of venous thromboembolic disease:**

a.   A ventilation-perfusion (V/Q) scan is a useful investigation if pulmonary embolism (PE) is suspected.
b.   A negative D-dimer in the context of low clinical probability reliably excludes PE.
c.   The incidence of venous thromboembolism in critically ill patients is around 65%.
d.   Patients with a confirmed pulmonary embolism secondary to cancer should be anticoagulated with low-molecular-weight heparin injections for at least 6 months.
e.   The Wells score can be used to guide further management and investigation.

48 In a patient with suspected iron overdose:

a.   Abdominal X-ray is a useful investigation.
b.   Activated charcoal should be offered if the patient presents within 1 hour of overdose.
c.   Endoscopic retrieval is recommended as a therapeutic option in the event of a large overdose and early presentation.
d.   Chelation therapy with desferrioxamine should be commenced immediately for patients with systemic features of toxicity.
e.   Early administration of intravenous proton pump inhibitors reduces the incidence of gastric scarring.

49 Regarding resourcing of intensive care units:

a.   ICUs staffed by intensivie care physicians have lower mortality rates than those staffed by non-intensivists.
b.   An intensivist:patient ratio of greater than 1:14 negatively impacts on patient care.
c.   Non-clinical inter-hospital transfer is associated with a two-fold increase in mortality.
d.   Patients admitted as an emergency to hospital over the weekend are twice as likely to die as those admitted on a weekday.
e.   Night-time discharge from intensive care has been shown to adversely influence mortality in a randomised controlled trial.

50 A 78-year-old male is admitted with community-acquired pneumonia and a CURB-65 score of 4. He has a good functional baseline. His chest X-ray shows a pleural effusion. Which of the following apply to him?

a.   *Legionella* should be routinely tested by sputum analysis.
b.   This patient should be reviewed for critical care admission.

c.   Oral antibiotics should be commenced immediately.
d.   Steroids are not recommended.
e.   If a pleural effusion has a pH of >7.2 on a diagnostic tap then formal chest drainage is indicated.

51 The 2012 Berlin definition of ARDS includes the following components:

a.   Continuous positive airway pressure (CPAP) or positive end-expiratory pressure (PEEP) >5cm H_2O.
b.   Murray score >2.
c.   Pulmonary artery occlusion pressure <15cm H_2O.
d.   pH <7.3.
e.   Evidence of a direct precipitant occurring within the preceding week.

52 Regarding the initial assessment and resuscitation of a patient with an acute upper GI bleed, the following statements apply:

a.   Platelet transfusion is not routinely indicated for patients who are not actively bleeding and are haemodynamically stable.
b.   Platelet transfusion is indicated in patients who are actively bleeding and have a platelet count of less than 80×10^9/L.
c.   Prothrombin complex concentrate should be given to patients who are taking warfarin and are actively bleeding.
d.   Fresh frozen plasma (FFP) should not be given unless the patient's prothrombin time (international normalised ratio [INR]) or activated partial thromboplastin time is greater than 2.5 times normal.
e.   Recombinant factor VIIa should be given early if available.

53 With regard to traumatic brain injury (TBI), the following interventions are supported by the Brain Trauma Foundation guidelines:

a.   Urgent prehospital triage direct to neuroscience centres.
b.   Therapeutic hypothermia for raised intracranial pressure refractory to first-line treatments.
c.   Hyperventilation to achieve hypocarbia.
d.   Osmotherapy in the presence of progressive neurological deterioration not attributable to extracranial causes.
e.   ICP monitoring in all patients with a Glasgow Coma Scale (GCS) of <8.

54 The following are true of severity of illness scoring systems in the critically ill patient:

a.   The Mortality Probability Model (MPM) can be used for individual prognostication.
b.   The selection of variables and their weights for the Acute Physiology and Chronic Health Evaluation II (APACHE II) score were derived through multiple logistic regression analysis.
c.   The Simplified Acute Physiology Score 2 (SAPS 2) score can be customised to a geographical region.
d.   An increase in the Sequential Organ Failure Assessment (SOFA) score during the first 48 hours in the ICU predicts a mortality rate of at least 50%.
e.   The Therapeutic Intervention Scoring System (TISS) assesses nursing workload.

55 Regarding viral encephalitis:

a.   It is commonly caused by the mumps virus.
b.   The disease usually affects the parietal lobes.
c.   CT of the brain is a useful investigation in suspected cases.
d.   *Herpes simplex* encephalitis has a mortality rate of up to 70% if untreated.

e. The most common presenting features are convulsions and hallucinations.

56 Giving your patient a FAST-HUG means paying strict attention to the following:

a. Airway concerns.
b. Falls prevention.
c. Humidification of ventilatory support.
d. Tracheostomy care.
e. Stress ulcer prophylaxis.

57 The following are principles regarding patient confidentiality and the management of confidential information in the UK:

a. Once an adult has died, their next of kin has the right to full access of the patient's medical records.
b. When a patient suffering from a genetically heritable disease has refused consent to disclosure, it is illegal to inform their next of kin.
c. Permission from the next of kin authorises disclosure of a patient's confidential medical records after their death.
d. Caldicott Guardians can authorise a treatment when the patient has refused to consent.
e. All NHS institutions must appoint a Caldicott Guardian.

58 The following are considered risk factors for aneurysmal subarachnoid haemorrhage:

a. Female gender.
b. Smoking history.
c. Ehlers-Danlos syndrome.
d. Pregnancy.
e. Hypotension.

59 When considering the diagnosis of ventilator-associated pneumonia (VAP) in a mechanically ventilated patient:

a. A CPIS score >6 has poor specificity for the diagnosis of VAP.
b. A VAP is defined as a hospital-acquired pneumonia occurring at any time point in a mechanically ventilated patient.
c. Ventilator care bundles may include the use of a low-volume low-pressure tapered cuff.
d. Use of endotracheal tubes with subglottic suction have level I evidence showing a reduced incidence of VAP.
e. Late VAP (>5 days) is most commonly caused by streptococcal or staphylococcal organisms.

60 Regarding the principles of medical ethics and consent:

a. Respect for a patient's autonomy means that an operation cannot be performed if a patient who has capacity refuses, even if it is deemed in the patient's best interest by the medical team.
b. Oral consent is explicit consent.
c. Non-maleficence retains primacy over autonomy as shown by blood and marrow donation.
d. In order to obtain informed consent the patient must be informed of all conceivable risks and benefits of the treatment.
e. Consent is needed from the next of kin to perform a procedure on an adult patient who lacks capacity.

Single best answer questions — select ONE answer from the five choices

61 A 66-year-old man presents with a 1-week history of diarrhoea and vomiting. He complains of severe back pain and generalised weakness, and is admitted to his local emergency department. He has reduced power in his lower limbs. He is ataxic, tachypnoeic and has double vision. He has a normal computed tomography (CT) of the brain. The next most appropriate test from the list below would be:

a. Urine dipstick.
b. Magnetic resonance imaging (MRI) of the brain.
c. Echocardiogram.
d. Spirometry.
e. Electroencephalography (EEG).

62 When managing nutritional status in a critically ill patient, which of the following statements is most accurate?

a. High gastric residual volumes should prompt prescription of a 7-day prokinetic regimen, following exclusion of obstructive causes.
b. Intravenous propofol infusion provides a significant proportion of daily calorie intake.
c. The Malnutrition Universal Screening Tool (MUST) is the gold standard for identifying malnourished patients.
d. Early parenteral nutrition should be commenced in patients who cannot meet calorific targets by enteral nutrition alone.
e. Early provision of glutamine antioxidant supplements for critically ill patients improves outcome.

Paper 1 Questions

63 A 17-year-old woman is brought into the emergency department by ambulance. She was found at home by her parents and admitted to taking 15g of paracetamol 10 hours previously. Activated charcoal was administered, an N-acetyl cysteine infusion commenced and 2L of crystalloid infused. Twenty-four hours after admission her GCS drops to 14 and bloods showed: pH 7.30, INR 5.7, serum potassium 4.4mmol/L, serum creatinine 290μmol/L and a lactate of 2.8mmol/L. She is not actively bleeding. The next management step should be:

a.   Bicarbonate infusion.
b.   Fresh frozen plasma.
c.   Immediate placement on the super-urgent liver transplant scheme.
d.   Renal replacement therapy.
e.   Administration of vitamin K.

64 A 78-year-old man has collapsed several hours ago and been found on the floor by the paramedics. He was found to be hypothermic at 32°C. His creatinine kinase is 10,000 IU. His serum potassium is 5mmol/L, urea is 20mmol/L and creatinine is 300μmol/L. The most important form of initial treatment should be:

a.   Intravenous infusion of warmed crystalloid.
b.   Active warming.
c.   Intravenous administration of mannitol 0.25-0.5g/kg.
d.   Intravenous furosemide.
e.   Urgent haemodialysis.

65 In the management of suspected hepatorenal syndrome in the critically ill patient, which of the following therapeutic options is likely to be most efficacious?

a. Transjugular intrahepatic portosystemic shunting (TIPSS).
b. Furosemide infusion titrated to a urine output of 0.5ml/kg/hr.
c. Human albumin infusion at a rate of 20g/day.
d. Intravenous terlipressin at a dose of 0.5-2mg 4-6-hourly.
e. Dopamine infusion for support of cardiac output.

66 A 58-year-old female is being managed on the critical care unit after a grade 3 subarachnoid haemorrhage (SAH). CT angiogram shows an aneurysm of the right middle cerebral artery. Forty-eight hours after the initial bleed she is awaiting surgical clipping when her GCS drops to 8 and she develops left-sided weakness. Transcranial Doppler ultrasonography shows a Lindegaard ratio of 2. Repeat CT shows hypodense fluid within the subarachnoid space and basal cisterns, and cresenteric temporal horns of the lateral ventricles. Her serum sodium level is 130mmol/L. The most likely cause for her deterioration is:

a. Vasospasm.
b. Rebleed.
c. Hydrocephalus.
d. Hyponatraemia.
e. Seizure.

67 A 28-year-old woman presents with intentional overdose of 30g of paracetamol. She has also ingested a large quantity of alcohol. Her GCS is initially normal but has fallen to 12 on review 8 hours into her admission. The most likely explanation for this is:

a. Cerebral oedema.
b. Cerebrovascular accident.
c. Intracerebral bleed.
d. Uraemia secondary to acute renal failure.
e. Hepatic encephalopathy secondary to decompensated chronic liver disease.

68 A patient arrives on the neurointensive care unit following a road traffic collision with resultant cervical spine fractures and cord injury. He undergoes urgent operative stabilisation the same day, and is extubatable. Three days later on clinical assessment, he is unable to move either leg but can flex both elbows and raise arms at the shoulder joint/shrug effectively when lying supine. He has absent sensation to a T2 dermatomal level with preservation around the sacral dermatomes S4/5 and sensation of deep anal pressure. Which of the following options best categorises the severity of his spinal cord injury?

a. ASIA impairment scale B.
b. ASIA impairment scale A.
c. ASIA impairment scale C.
d. MRC grading 1 left upper arm.
e. MRC grading 2 left upper arm.

69 A 77-year-old man is admitted to the intensive care unit following emergency repair of a ruptured abdominal aortic aneurysm. During the operation he received a 10-unit blood transfusion and was transferred to ICU intubated and ventilated, initially with minimal oxygen requirements. Twenty-four hours later his oxygen requirement has begun to increase. His P:F ratio is 28.3kPa and his chest X-ray shows new bibasal interstitial shadowing. An echocardiogram demonstrates good right and left ventricular function with an ejection fraction of 55%. His stroke volume variation is 14%. The most likely diagnosis is:

a. Acute lung injury (ALI).
b. Acute respiratory distress syndrome (ARDS).
c. Ventilator-associated pneumonia.
d. Transfusion-related acute lung injury.
e. Cardiogenic pulmonary oedema.

70 A 32-year-old male asthmatic is admitted to the emergency department with a 2-day history of increasing wheeze and shortness of breath. His HR is 115bpm, blood pressure is 120/60mmHg, respiratory rate is 28 breaths per minute with saturations of 92% on room air. He has a widespread expiratory wheeze refractory to his normal inhalers. The most appropriate next step in his management is:

a. Intubation and ventilation.
b. Intravenous magnesium 2g.
c. Urgent chest X-ray.
d. Back to back bronchodilator nebuliser therapy.
e. Intravenous hydrocortisone.

71 In a trauma patient with a high cervical spine injury, which of the following statements is most likely to be INCORRECT:

a. Progressive bradycardia and hypotension is most likely to be due to developing spinal shock.
b. In the hypotensive patient, haemorrhage should be sought and excluded as a matter of priority.
c. A mean arterial pressure of 90mmHg is advised to optimise cord perfusion.
d. Abdominal breathing is a sign of impending respiratory deterioration.
e. Flaccid areflexia and hypotonia can develop below the level of the lesion in the early phase, prior to the development of upper motor neurone signs.

72 A 57-year-old man is receiving pressure support ventilation via a tracheostomy for a ventilator-acquired pneumonia. He was admitted to the ICU following emergency left hemi-colectomy for perforated diverticular disease 10 days previously. He has an ileus, and a nasogastric tube *in situ* is on free drainage. He is becoming agitated, tachycardic and hypertensive but doesn't pose a threat to staff. His tracheostomy is patent and his capnography trace is normal. ECG shows sinus tachycardia (rate 121), normal axis, QTc 460ms. He has a fluctuating mental state, inattention and disorganised thinking, and a diagnosis of hyperactive delirium is made. What is the best pharmacological choice to manage his delirium?

a. Dexmedetomidine.
b. Propofol.
c. Haloperidol.
d. Midazolam.
e. Quetiapine.

73 A 54-year-old woman with a background of rheumatoid arthritis presents with progressive weakness. There is no preceding prodromal illness. She is globally weak with ptosis and fatigability. Gait is normal and there is no sensory loss. Her creatinine kinase is normal. The most likely diagnosis is:

a. Multiple sclerosis (MS).
b. Dermatomyositis.
c. Guillain-Barré syndrome (GBS).
d. Myasthenia gravis (MG).
e. Sub-acute degeneration of the spinal cord (SCD).

74 You receive a microbiology report on an intubated patient with severe acute respiratory failure and unilateral cavitating opacification on X-ray. The report suggests early growth from a recent bronchoalveolar lavage sample of Panton-Valentine leukocidin-producing *Staphylococcus aureus*. The patient is currently receiving co-amoxiclav for suspected community-acquired pneumonia. Clinically he is deteriorating with worsening septic shock and oxygenation. The best choice of antimicrobial therapy would be:

a. Intravenous flucloxacillin, clindamycin and meropenem.
b. Addition of intravenous immunoglobulin to the current regime.
c. Intravenous clindamycin, linezolid and rifampicin and consideration of intravenous immunoglobulin.
d. Intravenous vancomycin pending sensitivities.
e. Nebulised pentamidine with linezolid and consideration of intravenous immunoglobulin.

75 A 75-year-old patient is admitted to the ICU post-emergency laparotomy for colonic perforation. A Hartmann's procedure has been performed. Intra-operatively she has received 3L of Hartmann's solution and 500ml of gelofusine. She is now maintained intubated and ventilated with pressure support mode. She is becoming progressively more tachycardic and hypotensive. Which of the options would be the best indicator that a fluid bolus would be of benefit?

a. Central venous pressure of 6mmHg.
b. Stroke volume variation of 14%.
c. Pulmonary artery occlusion pressure of 10mmHg.
d. Passive leg raise increment in stroke volume of 12%.
e. Left ventricular end-diastolic diameter of 4cm in the parasternal long axis view.

76 A 60-year-old man with chronic obstructive pulmonary disease (COPD) presents with sudden onset shortness of breath to the emergency department. He has a respiratory rate of 24 breaths per minute. His saturations are 92% on room air. A 4cm right-sided pneumothorax is diagnosed on a plain chest X-ray. The most appropriate course of action is:

a. Simple needle aspiration of the pneumothorax with a 16G or 18G cannula.
b. Insertion of an intercostal chest drain on the right side.
c. High-flow oxygen therapy and close observation in a monitored area.
d. Emergency needle decompression on the right side.
e. Discharge home if there is no deterioration over a 4-hour period with return next day with repeat chest X-ray.

77 You are called to see a patient with a percutaneous tracheostomy *in situ* who has become distressed. He has desaturated to 85% and the nursing staff have placed him on a Water's circuit with an FiO_2 of 1.0 and removed the inner tube. The bag is barely shifting. The capnography trace is poor with no obvious waveform. He is sweaty and agitated. High-flow oxygen has been applied to the mouth and stoma. What is the most appropriate first step?

a.   Attempt to place a suction catheter down the tracheostomy.
b.   Bronchoscopy down the tracheostomy to assess position.
c.   Apply PEEP 5-10cm H_2O using the Water's circuit.
d.   Deflate the cuff of the tracheostomy tube.
e.   Remove the tracheostomy and attempt oral intubation.

78 A 55kg 81-year-old man suffers an acute myocardial infarction. Following coronary artery bypass grafting he is admitted to the cardiac intensive care unit. He is intubated and ventilated with no inotropic or vasopressor support. Cardiac output studies show: heart rate 115bpm, blood pressure is 131/78mmHg, central venous pressure 19mmHg, cardiac index 1.9L/min/m², pulmonary artery wedge pressure 24mmHg and systemic vascular resistance index 2800 dyne/s/cm⁵/m². His urine output is less than 20ml/hour, and his lactate is 6.1mmol/L. There is no evidence of tamponade on echocardiogram. The most appropriate medication would be:

a.   Milrinone.
b.   Dobutamine.
c.   Noradrenaline.
d.   Digoxin.
e.   Adrenaline.

79 A 67-year-old man is admitted having woken up at 0800 with a new hemiplegia of his right arm and leg. He was last seen well by his wife at 2200 the previous night. He has a history of high cholesterol but is not compliant with his medication. He smokes 20 cigarettes per day. A CT brain scan shows an acute left middle cerebral artery territory infarct. His blood pressure is 147/98mmHg. The following is the most important next step in his management:

a. Rapid transfer to local neurology stoke centre for urgent thrombolysis.
b. Clopidogrel 300mg for 7 days.
c. Aspirin 300mg for 14 days.
d. Intravenous labetolol aiming for a mean arterial pressure <90mmHg.
e. Discussion with a local neurosurgical centre.

80 A 59-year-old patient is referred following urgent assessment by the stroke team. He has attended with sudden onset visual disturbance, followed by decreased GCS and left-sided hemiparesis. CT has demonstrated a right-sided middle cerebral artery thrombus. He was unfortunately outside the window for thrombolysis, but has been managed on the stroke unit with antiplatelet therapy. It is now 48 hours post-event and his GCS has continued to deteriorate, from 12 yesterday to 7 today. Which of the following options is most likely to reduce mortality?

a. Interventional radiology and clot retrieval.
b. External ventricular drain insertion.
c. Delayed thrombolysis.
d. Decompressive hemicraniectomy.
e. Placement of an intracranial pressure bolt and titrated medical therapy to achieve an ICP <20mmHg.

81. A 44-year-old patient with a history of alcohol excess is mechanically ventilated on the ICU following a traumatic brain injury. He develops chest sepsis and multi-organ dysfunction with acute kidney injury and deranged liver function, and requires a noradrenaline infusion to support his blood pressure. Following a sedation hold he becomes agitated and requires re-sedation. Observations during the sedation hold include blood pressure 90/50mmHg, heart rate 120bpm (sinus tachycardia), intracranial pressure 15mmHg. The most appropriate sedative regime would be:

a.   Morphine and midazolam infusions.
b.   Propofol and fentanyl infusions.
c.   Propofol and remifentanil infusions.
d.   Dexmedetomidine infusion.
e.   Thiopentone infusion.

82. A 67-year-old male with a background of alcohol excess is admitted to the emergency department. He has a brief tonic-clonic seizure and is moved to the resuscitation room. He is post-ictal but rousable to voice. Finger-prick blood sugar is 3.5mmol/L. The first intervention should be:

a.   Chlordiazepoxide 10-20mg.
b.   Intravenous vitamin supplementation.
c.   Intravenous glucose 10-20g.
d.   Intravenous phenytoin loading.
e.   Urgent CT brain scan.

83 A 24-year-old patient arrives on the unit following a traumatic brain injury, with florid frontal and right temporal contusions on CT imaging. He went directly to theatre from admission for insertion of a Codman ICP probe and an external ventricular drain (EVD), which is currently at 10cm and draining clear cerebrospinal fluid (CSF) well. He has no other medical injuries. Twenty-four hours following admission his ICP rises to 30mmHg and plateaus. Tier 1 neuroprotection is ongoing. His $ETCO_2$ is currently 4kPa and his MAP is 95mmHg. His EVD continues to drain clear CSF. Which of the following options to manage his intracranial hypertension is the most appropriate next step?

a. Administration of 3% hypertonic saline.
b. Hyperventilation to an $ETCO_2$ of 3kPa.
c. Decompressive hemicraniectomy.
d. Removal of the external ventricular drain.
e. Bolus of 500ml 4.5% human albumin solution to increase intravascular colloid pressure.

84 A 55-year-old man is admitted to a major trauma centre following a motor vehicle collision. He is taken to theatre for damage control surgery. The massive transfusion protocol is activated. Intra-operatively, he receives 8 units of packed red cells, 8 units of fresh frozen plasma and 8 pooled doses of platelets. The surgeon has clamped a bleeding vessel but reports that the surgical field continues to ooze. A thromboelastogram is performed and shows: R-time 10 minutes, K-time 3 minutes, angle 62°, maximum amplitude 71mm, clot lysis at 60 minutes 11%. Given these results, what is the most appropriate blood product/medication to administer to improve haemostasis?

a.   Fresh frozen plasma.
b.   Cryoprecipitate.
c.   Platelets.
d.   Recombinant factor VII.
e.   Tranexamic acid.

85   A 66-year-old man is admitted with a 2-week history of intermittent left shoulder pain. He has a mild cough. He is a smoker but otherwise fit and well. He suddenly becomes breathless in the early hours with blood-stained sputum. He is hypoxic with a paO_2 of 7.0kPa on 15L/min of oxygen. A chest X-ray shows diffuse pulmonary infiltrates. A 12-lead ECG shows sinus tachycardia with lateral T-wave inversion. His blood pressure is 134/98mmHg. The next step in his management should be:

a.   Urgent thrombolysis with fibrinolytic agent.
b.   Continuous positive airway pressure (CPAP).
c.   Intra-aortic balloon pump (IABP).
d.   Transfer for primary coronary intervention (PCI).
e.   Blood culture and early administration of intravenous antibiotics.

86   When using intra-aortic balloon (IABP) counterpulsation to treat cardiogenic shock, the intervention will achieve all of the following EXCEPT:

a.   Improvement in coronary perfusion.
b.   Increase left ventricular stroke work index.
c.   Reduction in afterload.
d.   Increase in diastolic blood pressure.
e.   Increase in renal blood flow.

87 An 82-year-old female has been intubated and ventilated on the ICU for the past 6 days following emergency surgery for a ruptured abdominal aortic aneurysm. Her oxygen requirements increase and she becomes tachypnoeic. She develops an increased load of non-purulent secretions. She develops a tachycardia and spikes a temperature of 39.1°C. On auscultation there is decreased air entry and some crackles bibasally with dullness to percussion at the right base. Bloods show an FiO_2/PaO_2 of 34kPa and serum white cell count 13 x $10^9/L$ with 55% band forms. Chest X-ray shows new shadowing in the lower zones with loss of the right hemi-diaphragm. What is the most appropriate diagnosis?

a.   Pulmonary embolism.
b.   Pleural effusion.
c.   Ventilator-associated pneumonia.
d.   Acute respiratory distress syndrome.
e.   Pulmonary oedema.

88 A 57-year-old man with alcohol-related liver disease (Child-Pugh Class B) is admitted in the early hours with an upper gastrointestinal bleed and gross ascites. He is intubated and ventilated to facilitate an urgent endoscopy which shows three oesophageal varices which are banded. The next morning he fails a spontaneous breathing trial and is resedated. The most appropriate course of action would be:

a.   Insertion of an ascitic drain with 100ml 20% albumin cover for every 3L of ascites drained.
b.   Intravenous terlipressin.

c. Trial of extubation onto non-invasive ventilation.
d. An ascitic drain with 100ml 4.5% albumin for every 3L ascites drained.
e. Start spironolactone and repeat spontaneous breathing trial after 24 hours.

89 A patient is referred to the intensive care unit with breathlessness and confirmed H1N1 influenza. Currently she is saturating at 97% on an FiO_2 of 0.35, with a pulse of 120 and a temperature of 39.5°C. Her respiratory rate is 32. The medical team caring for her believe she has deteriorated over the last 12 hours. Which of the following facts would most influence your decision to move her to a critical care environment?

a. She is elderly.
b. She is obese.
c. She is pregnant.
d. She has not received oseltamivir since hospital admission.
e. She is lymphopenic.

90 A 45-year-old male is admitted with fever, rigors and a heart murmur. He is an intravenous drug user. A clinical diagnosis of infective endocarditis is made. Which of the following is the most likely causative organism?

a. *Streptococcus bovis.*
b. *Candida albicans.*
c. *Streptococcus viridans.*
d. *Staphylococcus aureus.*
e. *Chlamydia psittaci.*

Paper 1
Answers

1   F, F, T, F, F

Guillain-Barré syndrome (GBS) affects individuals of all ages, although there is a bimodal tendency towards young adults and the elderly. There is a slight male preponderance. The disease usually affects children with less clinical severity. The majority of cases of GBS occur within a month of either a respiratory or gastrointestinal infection. The commonest pathogen is *Campylobacter jejuni*. Many other organisms such as Epstein-Barr virus, *Mycoplasma pneumoniae* and *Cytomegalovirus* may also be implicated. Miller Fisher is a variant of the disease. Clinical features of this subtype include ataxia, areflexia and ophthalmoplegia, which may be accompanied by limb weakness, ptosis and facial/bulbar palsy.

1. Richards KJC, Cohen AT. Guillain-Barré syndrome. *Br J Anaesth CEPD Rev* 2003; 3(2): 46-9.

2   T, T, F, T, F

Initial hypotensive resuscitation is recommended for both blunt and penetrating trauma during early resuscitation within the emergency department. European guidelines recommend the use of desmopressin, but advise consideration of rFVIIa only when platelets have been corrected to >50 x 10^9/L. The same guidelines have also recently adjusted recommendations to advise against the use of aprotinin, given the strong evidence base for tranexamic acid. A recent meta-analysis confirms the increased risk of pre-injury warfarin use in blunt traumatic brain injury (TBI).

1. Spahn DR, Bouillon B, Cerny V, *et al*. Management of bleeding and coagulopathy following major trauma: an updated European guideline. *Crit Care* 2013; 17(2): R76.
2. Batchelor JS, Grayson A. A meta-analysis to determine the effect of anticoagulation on mortality in patients with blunt head trauma. *Br J Neurosurg* 2012; 26(4): 525-30.

3   T, T, T, F, T

Most drugs undergo metabolism, usually to less active species. Phase I metabolism includes oxidation, reduction and hydrolysis; phase II includes glucuronidation, sulphation, acetylation, methylation and glycination. Most phase I and II reactions occur in the liver; however, some drugs undergo non-organ metabolism. Esmolol is hydrolysed by non-specific plasma esterases. Atracurium undergoes Hoffmann degradation in the plasma — spontaneous breakdown in a pH- and temperature-dependent manner. Inhaled nitric oxide is rapidly broken down in the blood and blood vessel walls. It binds to oxyhaemoglobin, forming methaemaglobin and nitrate. Propofol undergoes hepatic metabolism, 40% is conjugated to a glucuronide and 60% to a quinol, which is excreted in the urine as inactive glucuronides and sulphates. Adrenaline is metabolised by mitochondrial monamine oxidase (MAO) and catechol O-methyl transferase (COMT) within the liver, kidney and blood to the inactive 3-methoxy-4hydroxymandelic acid and metadrenaline which is conjugated with glucuronic acid and sulphates, both of which are excreted in the urine.

1. Peck TE, Williams M. *Pharmacology for Anaesthesia and Intensive Care*. London, UK: Greenwich Medical Media, 2002.

4   F, F, T, F, F

A raised $PaCO_2$ is a sign of a 'near-fatal' asthma attack. A peak expiratory flow rate (PEFR) <33% predicted is associated with a life-threatening acute exacerbation. A PaO_2 of <8kPa is a life-threatening sign according to the guideline as is a silent chest and arrhythmias. An inability to complete sentences in one breath is a sign of acute severe asthma.

1. British Thoracic Society. British guideline on the management of asthma: a national clinical guideline 101.
2. http://www.sign.ac.uk/guidelines/fulltext/101/index.html (accessed 30th September 2014).

5   T, T, F, T, T

Fresh frozen plasma (FFP) is usually administered at a dose of 10-15ml/kg initially. Cryoprecipitate is manufactured by thawing FFP at 4°C and removing the precipitated layer. This 'cryoprecipitate' is then centrifuged and re-suspended in 20-40ml of plasma. It is a product rich in Factor VIII and fibrinogen, thus it is often used in bleeding with hypofibrinogenaemia.

Desmopressin has antidiuretic properties and can also promote haemostasis, by inducing the release of vWF from endothelial storage sites, improving platelet adhesion and increasing plasma activity of Factor VIII.

Hypothermia can be disastrous in a patient with massive haemorrhage, forming one side of the lethal triad alongside acidosis and coagulopathy. There is evidence to suggest a reduction in enzyme kinetics by a third with a measurable deficit in the prothrombin and activated partial thromboplastin time at temperatures of 33°C.

1. Ridley S, Taylor B, Gunning K. Medical management of bleeding in critically ill patients. *Contin Educ Anaesth Crit Care Pain* 2007; 7(4): 116-21.
2. Johnston TD, Chen Y, Reed RL. Functional equivalence of hypothermia to specific clotting factor deficiencies. *J Trauma* 1994; 37: 413-7.

6   F, F, T, F, T

Affinity refers to how well the drug binds to its receptor and activity refers to the magnitude of the effect once the drug has bound. An agonist has receptor affinity and activity whereas an antagonist has receptor affinity but no activity. Full agonists are drugs that are able to generate a maximal response from the receptor, partial agonists have only moderate intrinsic activity and produce a submaximal effect compared with a full agonist; by definition increasing the dose cannot achieve a maximal effect. Inverse agonists bind to the receptor but exert an effect opposite to that of the endogenous agonist. Flumazenil is an antagonist. The effects of a reversible antagonist can be overcome by increasing the concentration of the agonist. Increasing the concentration of an agonist will not overcome the effects of an irreversible antagonist.

1.   Peck TE, Williams M. *Pharmacology for Anaesthesia and Intensive Care.* London, UK: Greenwich Medical Media, 2002.

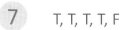

7   T, T, T, T, F

Hepatorenal syndrome (HRS) is frequently misdiagnosed. Distinguishing between HRS and both pre-renal failure and acute tubular necrosis (ATN) may be difficult. The following are the diagnostic criteria:

* Cirrhosis with ascites.
* Creatinine >133µmol/L.
* Absence of shock.
* Absence of hypovolaemia (no response to diuretic withdrawal and albumin volume expansion).
* No nephrotoxic drugs.
* No parenchymal renal disease (normal ultrasound and urinary sediment protein <0.5g/day).
* <50 red blood cells per high-powered field on microscopy.

Two subtypes, 1 and 2, are traditionally recognised, but more recently subtypes 3 and 4 have been identified. The prognosis in Type 1 HRS is poor, with a median untreated survival of 2 weeks. Type 2 HRS has a median survival of 6 months in keeping with the slower renal decline. The presence of HRS in an organ donor does not preclude transplantation of their kidneys to a patient without liver disease. In liver cirrhosis there is a vasodilated splanchnic circulation due to overproduction of nitric oxide (NO). Terlipressin is a powerful vasopressin V1 receptor agonist which causes systemic vasoconstriction and raises blood pressure. It is long-acting and can be given as peripheral boluses.

1. World Federation of Societies of Anaesthesiologists. Lynch G. Hepatorenal syndrome. Anaesthesia Tutorial of the Week 240, September 2011. www.aagbi.org/education/educational-resources/tutorial-week (accessed 26th February 2015).
2. http://www.frca.co.uk/Documents/240%20Hepatorenal%20syndrome.pdf (accessed 30th September 2014).

8   F, F, F, T, T

The use of suxamethonium is challenging in patients with neuromuscular disorders. Key points to remember include relative resistance to depolarisation in myasthenia gravis, often requiring an increased dosage, and the development of extrajunctional receptors in many of the myotonias, leading to extensive depolarisation and potentially fatal hyperkalaemia with the use of depolarising neuromuscular blockade. In addition, there are disease-specific aspects of non-depolarising neuromuscular blockade that should be noted, including the relative sensitivity in conditions such as Guillain-Barré syndrome. If required, dose reduction to 10-20% should be considered in addition to ongoing monitoring of blockade.

1. Marsh S, Ross N, Pittard A. Neuromuscular disorders and anaesthesia part 1. *Contin Educ Anaesth Crit Care Pain* 2011; 11(4): 115-8.
2. Marsh S, Pittard A. Neuromuscular disorders and anaesthesia part 2. *Contin Educ Anaesth Crit Care Pain* 2011; 11(4): 119-23.

9   F, F, T, F, F

Guidelines vary, but in general enteral feeding is deemed to be successful if feed is running at greater than or equal to 40ml/hr with 4-hourly aspirates totalling <250ml — many experts would consider even higher volume aspirates to be consistent with successful enteral feeding. When enteral feeding is unsuccessful, parenteral nutrition should be considered. Studies have shown that survival of critically ill patients is best among patients who receive 33-66% of estimated nutritional needs. Parenteral nutrition is usually administered through a dedicated lumen of a central venous catheter or through a peripherally inserted central catheter. Low osmolality feeds can, however, be administered through a peripheral venous line. Protein is administered to replace nitrogen losses and prevent further skeletal muscle breakdown; calculation of actual nitrogen balance is difficult so administration of 0.13-0.24g/kg/day of nitrogen is suggested. This usually equates to 1g/kg/day of protein. Trace elements are not present in commercially produced parenteral nutrition solutions for stability reasons and therefore must be prescribed separately.

1.   Macdonald K, Page K, Brown L, Bryden D. Parenteral nutrition in critical care. *Contin Educ Anaesth Crit Care Pain* 2013; 13(1): 1-5.
2.   National Institute for Health and Care Excellence, National Collaborating Centre for Acute Care. Nutrition support in adults. NICE clinical guideline 32. London, UK: NICE, 2006. www.nice.org.uk (accessed 25th February 2015).

10   T, F, F, T, F

Some of the medications reported to cause exacerbations of myasthenia gravis (MG) include the following:

* Antibiotics — macrolides, fluoroquinolones, aminoglycosides, tetracycline, and chloroquine.
* Anti-dysrhythmic agents — β-blockers, calcium channel blockers, quinidine, lignocaine, procainamide, and trimethaphan.
* Miscellaneous — diphenylhydantoin, lithium, chlorpromazine, muscle relaxants, levothyroxine, adrenocorticotropic hormone (ACTH), and, paradoxically, corticosteroids.

1.   World Federation of Societies of Anaesthesiologists. Banerjee A. Anaesthesia and myasthenia gravis. Anaesthesia Tutorial of the Week 122, 15th December 2008. www.aagbi.org/education/educational-resources/tutorial-week (accessed 26th February 2015).
2.   http//www.anaesthesiauk.com/Documents/122%20Myasthenia%20Gravis.pdf (accessed 20th August 2014).

11 F, F, F, F, F

A peak expiratory flow rate (PEFR) of <33% defines life-threatening asthma. There is limited evidence to support the use of aminophylline and British Thoracic Society guidelines suggest consideration only. The 3MG trial showed only a minor reduction in patient-reported breathlessness with the use of IV magnesium, with no effect on morbidity or need for invasive ventilation. Ketamine should be dosed at 1-2mg/kg. It has bronchodilator properties that make it an attractive induction agent for asthmatic patients. Fluid administration should be generous due to the common reduction in preload, as a result of gas trapping and raised intrathoracic pressure often limiting venous return.

1. Turner S, Paton J, Higgins B, Douglas G. British guidelines on the management of asthma: what's new for 2011? *Thorax* 2011; 66(12): 1104-5.
2. Goodacre S, Cohen J, Bradburn M, *et al*. Intravenous or nebulised magnesium sulphate versus standard therapy for severe acute asthma (3Mg trial): a double-blind, randomised controlled trial. *Lancet Respir Med* 2012; 1(4): 293-300.

12 F, T, T, F, F

Selective digestive tract decontamination (SDD) was first used in 1982. It is a prophylactic strategy to prevent nosocomial infections from potentially pathogenic micro-organisms of the oropharyngeal and intestinal tracts. Approximately 15 potentially pathogenic micro-organisms (PPMs) cause the majority of infections in the ICU. SDD is 'selective' because it targets aerobes and yeast only, with a sparing effect for anaerobic bacteria. Most protocols include a short (4-day) course of IV antibiotics for primary endogenous infections caused by PPMs; intragastric and oral (non-absorbable) antimicrobials throughout the ICU stay to control secondary endogenous infections due to PPMs acquired in the ICU; a high level of hygiene to prevent exogenous infections; and surveillance cultures of the respiratory tract and rectum to monitor decontamination efficacy and emergence of SDD-resistant pathogens. SDD has not been incorporated into standard practice in many healthcare systems in part due to concerns regarding antibiotic resistance, although there is limited evidence that this is the case.

1. Stoutenbeek CP, van Saene HKF, Miranda DR, Zandstra DF. The effect of selective decontamination of the digestive tract on colonization and infection rate in multiple trauma patients. *Intensive Care Med* 1984; 10(4): 185-92.
2. Bonten MJM. Selective digestive tract decontamination - will it prevent infection with multidrug-resistant Gram-negative pathogens but still be applicable in institutions where methicillin-resistant *Staphylococcus aureus* and vancomycin-resistant enterococci are endemic? *Clin Infect Dis* 2006; 43: S70-4.
3. Price R, MacLennan G, Glen J. Selective digestive or oropharyngeal decontamination and topical oropharyngeal chlorhexidine for prevention of death in general intensive care: systematic review and network meta-analysis. *Br Med J* 2014; 348: g2197.

13   F, T, T, T, F

Nephrotic syndrome is kidney disease with proteinuria, hypoalbuminemia, and oedema. Nephrotic-range proteinuria is 3g/24 hours or more. Metabolic consequences of the nephrotic syndrome include the following:

* Infection.
* Hypovolaemia.
* Hyperlipidaemia and atherosclerosis.
* Hypercoagulability.
* Hypocalcaemia and other bone abnormalities.

Infection is a major concern in nephrotic syndrome; patients have an increased susceptibility to infection with *Streptococcus pneumoniae*, *Haemophilus influenzae*, *Escherichia coli*, and other Gram-negative organisms. *Varicella* infection is also common. The most common infectious complications are bacterial sepsis, peritonitis, pneumonia and cellulitis.

Explanations for susceptibility to infection include: immunosuppressive therapy; urinary immunoglobulin loss; loss of complement factors with a role in opsonisation; protein deficiency, and reduction in leucocyte bactericidal activity.

Hypovolaemia is caused by hypoalbuminaemia which decreases the plasma oncotic pressure, with a consequent decrease in circulating blood volume. Hypovolaemia usually occurs only when the patient's serum albumin level is less than 1.5 g/dL.

Hyperlipidaemia may be considered a typical feature of nephrotic syndrome, rather than a complication. It relates to hypoproteinaemia and low serum oncotic pressure, with resultant hepatic protein synthesis as a reactive mechanism.

Atherosclerotic vascular disease has a higher prevalence in persons with nephrotic syndrome and thus myocardial infarction can occur.

Venous thrombosis and pulmonary embolism are well-recognised complications of nephrotic syndrome. Hypercoagulability is due to urinary loss of antithrombin III and plasminogen (anticoagulant factors), along with an increase in clotting factors, especially Factors I, VII, VIII, and X.

Hypocalcaemia is common in nephrotic syndrome but it is usually caused by a low serum albumin level rather than a low ionised calcium result. However, low bone density and abnormal bone histology are indeed reported with nephrotic syndrome, and may be explained by urinary losses of vitamin D-binding proteins.

1.   Cohen EP, Vatuman B. Nephrotic syndrome. http//www.emedicine.medscape.com/article/244631 (accessed August 13th 2014).

14   T, T, F, T, T

Much effort has been put into the development of prognostic models for traumatic brain injury (TBI) and large datasets within clinical trials have facilitated this. The MRC CRASH trial, for example, performed logistic regression to assess for key prognostic components at presentation, within a large cohort of TBI patients. An online calculator has been developed and is freely available. The model includes age, GCS, pupillary reaction, injury sustained within a low-middle income country, extracranial injury and CT findings. The presence of sensory deficit plays no role.

Other models exist such as the IMPACT calculator, which again can be found online. This model was derived from a cohort of 11 studies including >8000 patients and validated within the CRASH dataset of >6000 patients. The model has been adjusted to incorporate the impact of secondary insults on prognosis, and thus includes serum glucose, anaemia, hypotension and hypoxia.

1.   Perel P, Arango M, Clayton T, *et al*. Predicting outcome after traumatic brain injury: practical prognostic models based on large cohort of international patients. *Br Med J* 2008; 336(7641): 425-9.
2.   http://www.trialscoordinatingcentre.lshtm.ac.uk/Risk%20calculator/index.html (accessed 26th February 2015).
3.   http://www.tbi-impact.org/?p=impact/calc (accessed 26th February 2015).
4.   Steyerberg EW, Mushkudiani N, Perel P, *et al*. Predicting outcome after traumatic brain injury: development and international validation of prognostic scores based on admission characteristics. *PLOS (Medicine)* 2008; 5(8): e165.

15   F, F, F, T, T

Ventricular assist devices (VADs) are used to support the failing heart, either as a bridge to recovery, a bridge to transplant or as destination therapy. VADs are either used as short-term therapy, where the unit is predominantly extracorporeal, or as long-term therapy, where the device is predominantly intracorporeal. There are no limits to the length of time a VAD can be used for. The devices can be used to support the right side of the heart (RVAD, taking blood from the right atrium and injecting it into the main pulmonary artery), the left side of the heart (LVAD, taking blood from the left atrium and injecting it into the ascending aorta) or both sides (BIVAD). First-generation devices produce pulsatile flow whereas second- and third-generation devices produce continuous, non-pulsatile flow. This reduces the pump size and the need for external venting. Aortic insufficiency must be identified or excluded before an LVAD is inserted. After LVAD insertion the gradient between the mean arterial pressure and left ventricular end-diastolic pressure increases; this worsens aortic regurgitation and causes recirculation of the blood through the VAD, therefore, decreasing cardiac output. Mitral regurgitation often improves after LVAD insertion due to decompression of the LV. All VADs require anticoagulation and the inability to tolerate anticoagulation is a contraindication to insertion.

1. Harris P, Kuppurao L. Ventricular assist devices. *Contin Educ Anaesth Crit Care Pain* 2012; 12(3): 145-51.

16   T, F, F, T, F

Meningitis is a relatively rare complication of lumbar puncture (LP). It is contraindicated in patients with a suspected spinal epidural abscess. Suspected bacteraemia is NOT a contraindication to LP. Antiplatelet therapy with aspirin and non-steroidal anti-inflammatory agents has not been demonstrated to be clearly associated with increased bleeding after LP. It is recommended to suspend therapy, when possible, prior to elective LP. The antiplatelet effect of aspirin will take around a week to wear off. Performing an LP is not recommended in patients with coagulation defects who are actively bleeding, have severe thrombocytopaenia (e.g. platelet counts <50,000 to 80,000/μL), or an International Normalised Ratio (INR) >1.4, without correcting the underlying abnormalities. Discussion with a local haematologist is advised if in doubt.

1. Johnson KS, Sexton DJ. Lumbar puncture: technique, indications, contraindications, and complications in adults, 2013. *UpToDate*. http://www.uptodate.com/contents/lumbar-puncture-technique-indications-contraindications-and-complications-in-adults (accessed 28th July 2014).

17   T, T, F, F, T

Ocular nerve sheath diameter has been demonstrated to correlate well against invasive intracranial pressure monitoring when specific cut-offs are utilised, and in real time. As such it is a useful tool in the early stages of traumatic brain injury and can guide therapy prior to the placement of definitive intracranial pressure (ICP) monitoring. An ocular nerve sheath diameter of >5mm predicts ICP of >20mmHg with a sensitivity and specificity of around 90%.

An external ventricular drain allows removal of cerebrospinal fluid, which can dramatically reduce intracranial pressure secondary to volume expansion within the skull.

On a standard intracranial pressure waveform, P1 represents systolic contraction, P2 represents cerebral compliance and P3 represents the dichrotic notch. Cerebral blood flow increases in response to hypoxia and causes a profound elevation in ICP.

Lundberg waves are a separate entity looking at the change in ICP over a prolonged period of time. A-waves are steep increases in ICP lasting for 5-10 minutes at a time. They are always pathological and usually represent early brain herniation. B-waves are slow oscillations every 1-2 minutes, representing potential vasospasm, and C-waves are physiologically normal fast oscillations, occurring 4-8 times per minute.

1. Kimberly HH, Shah S, Marill K, Noble V. Correlation of optic nerve sheath diameter with direct measurement of intracranial pressure. *Acad Emerg Med* 2008; 15(2): 201-4.
2. Geeraerts T, Merceron S, Benhamou D, *et al*. Non-invasive assessment of intracranial pressure using ocular sonography in neurocritical care patients. *Intensive Care Med* 2008; 34(11): 2062-7.

18   T, T, F, T, T

Total positive end-expiratory pressure (PEEP) is an increase in the end-expiratory pressure. It is made up of intrinsic PEEP (PEEPi, an increase in the static recoil pressure of the respiratory system, usually due to airflow obstruction) and extrinsic PEEP (PEEPe, positive pressure applied to the expiratory limb of the circuit). During spontaneous ventilation, work must be done to overcome PEEPi before airflow can occur. Applying PEEPe less than the PEEPi will reduce this elastic work required to initiate airflow. PEEP maintains recruitment of collapsed lung, increases functional residual capacity and minimises intra-pulmonary shunt, thus improving oxygenation. PEEP reduces venous return and therefore cardiac output; oxygen delivery may therefore fall despite an improvement in oxygenation. PEEP must be titrated to achieve a balance between oxygenation and haemodynamic optimisation.

Volume-controlled ventilation (VCV) delivers a constant flow and pressure increases linearly until a peak pressure is achieved. Pressure-controlled ventilation (PCV) produces a decelerating flow pattern and a constant pressure is delivered. The peak pressure (Ppk) achieved during VCV is dependent on the elastic and resistive properties of the respiratory system. When an end-inspiratory pause is added, airways and tissue resistance dissipate and the pressure falls to reach a plateau pressure (Pplat). In PCV this resistance dissipates during inspiration so that Ppk and Pplat are equal, and thus an end-inspiratory pause is not usually required to measure Pplat. Compliance is the change in volume per unit change in pressure and elastance is the inverse of compliance. Static compliance is measured when there is no airflow and dynamic where airflow is present.

Static compliance	Vt/(Pplat-PEEPtotal)
Dynamic compliance	Vt/(Ppk-PEEPtotal)
Static elastance	(Pplat-PEEPtotal)/Vt
Dynamic elastance	(Ppk-PEEPtotal)/Vt

1.   Bersten AD, Soni N. *Oh's Intensive Care Manual*, 6th ed. Philadelphia, USA: Butterworth Heinemann, Elsevier, 2009.

19   T, F, T, T, F

Multiple scoring systems directly applicable to critical care patients have been introduced and developed over the last 30 years. They allow an assessment of the severity of disease and provide a means of predicting consequent mortality within a cohort, but not for individual patients. Examples include the APACHE, SOFA, MDM, Simplified Acute Physiology Score (SAPS) and Multiple Organ Dysfunction Score (MODS). The CT Calcium Score Tool has been developed to help clarify the role CT calcium scoring can play in the exclusion of anginal disease in people presenting with chest pain of suspected cardiac origin. The Glasgow-Blatchford Score is used to risk stratify patients with upper gastrointestinal bleeding at first presentation and has little applicability to those who are critically ill.

1.   Bouch DC, Thompson JP. Severity scoring systems in the critically ill. *Contin Educ Anaesth Crit Care Pain* 2008; 8(5): 181-5.
2.   National Institute for Health and Care Excellence. CT calcium scoring. NICE clinical guideline 95. London, UK: NICE, July 2010. www.nice.org.uk (accessed 25th February 2015).

20 T, F, T, T, T

A superiority RCT aims to demonstrate a benefit in the primary outcome of an interventional treatment over the control arm. Hence, the null hypothesis is usually that no difference exists between the two groups.

The Protocolized Care for Early Septic Shock (ProCESS) trial has recently demonstrated no benefit to protocolised therapy in sepsis over standard care, the Targered Temperature Management (TTM) trial demonstrated no benefit in therapeutic hypothermia to 33°C over 36°C after cardiac arrest, the Vasopressin and Septic Shock Trial (VASST) demonstrated no benefit to vasopressin in septic shock in addition to low-dose noradrenaline, and the Oscillation in ARDS (OSCAR) trial showed no improvement with high-frequency oscillatory ventilation in patients with severe acute respiratory distress syndrome (ARDS) compared to standard care.

The Proning Severe ARDS Patients (PROSEVA) trial noted a reduction in mortality for those patients with severe ARDS placed in the prone position within the early stages of care and as such rejected the null hypothesis.

1. The ProCESS Investigators. A randomized trial of protocol-based care for early septic shock. *N Engl J Med* 2014; 370: 1683-93.
2. Nielsen N, Wetterslev J, Cronberg T, *et al*. Targeted temperature management at 33 degrees versus 36 degrees after cardiac arrest. *N Engl J Med* 2013; 369: 2197-206.
3. Russell JA, Walley KR, Singer J, *et al*. Vasopressin versus norepinephrine infusion in patients with septic shock. *N Engl J Med* 2008; 358(9): 877-87.
4. Young D, Lamb SE, Shah S, *et al*. High-frequency oscillation for acute respiratory distress syndrome. *N Engl J Med* 2013; 68(9): 806-13.
5. Guerin C, Reignier J, Richard JC, *et al*. Prone positioning in severe acute respiratory distress syndrome. *N Engl J Med* 2013; 368(23): 2159-68.

21 T, T, F, T, F

Therapeutic plasma exchange is a procedure in which large volumes of plasma are removed from the patient and replaced with some form of replacement fluid. The most commonly used replacement fluid is 4.5% human albumin in physiological saline, although the use of fresh frozen plasma is preferential in a limited number of disorders. Plasma exchange is most useful for autoimmune and immunoproliferative diseases, including thrombotic thrombocytopaenia purpura (TTP). Its use in TTP has reduced mortality rates from over 90% to 10-20%. Whilst central access is frequently used, up to 67% of therapeutic plasma exchange procedures can be completed successfully with peripheral venous access. Bulk removal of plasma removes both clotting factors and inhibitors of coagulation. Coagulation may become temporarily deranged. Theoretically, the removal of inhibitors of coagulation could predispose to thrombosis, but this has not been definitively demonstrated. Paraesthesia related to hypocalcaemia resulting from the use of citrate anticoagulant is the most common reaction seen as a result of therapeutic plasma exchange.

1. Winters JL. Plasma exchange: concepts, mechanism, and an overview of the American Society for Apheresis guidelines. *Haematology* 2012; 2012: 7-12.
2. Scully M, Hunt BJ, Benjamin S, *et al*. Guidelines on the diagnosis and management of thrombotic thrombocytopenic purpura and other thrombotic microangiopathies. *Br J Haem* 2012; 158: 323-5.

22   T, F, F, T, F

In the absence of haemorrhagic shock, Kidney Disease: Improving Global Outcomes (KDIGO) international consensus guidelines suggest using isotonic crystalloids rather than colloids (albumin or starches) as the initial management for expansion of intravascular volume in patients at risk for acute kidney injury (AKI) or with AKI. In critically ill patients, they suggest insulin therapy targeting plasma glucose 110-149mg/dL (6.1-8.3mmol/L). The guidelines also suggest providing nutrition preferentially via the enteral route in patients with AKI. The low-dose dopamine and oral or intravenous N-acetyl cysteine (NAC) for the prevention of post-surgical AKI are not recommended.

1. Kidney Disease Improving Global Outcomes (KDIGO) clinical practice guideline for acute kidney injury. Official journal of The International Society of Nephrology. *Kidney Int* Suppl 2012; 2(1): 8-12.

23 T, F, T, T, F

The CRASH trials are slightly confusing, as they are not all about traumatic brain injury and the CRASH acronym stands for something different in each trial. The original CRASH (Corticosteroid Randomisation After Significant Head injury) trial looked at steroids in head injury. CRASH 2 (Clinical Randomisation of an Antifibrinolytic in Significant Haemorrhage) examined the use of tranexamic acid for major trauma within a multicentre international cohort, then published a subgroup analysis of a nested pilot which suggested that tranexamic acid may reduce the development of intracranial haematoma expansion. As such, CRASH 3 is currently recruiting to look at the use of tranexamic acid specifically for isolated TBI.

There is now level I evidence against steroid use in TBI and as such they are not recommended within the latest TBI consensus guidelines.

1.   Edwards P, Arango M, Balica L, et al. Final results of MRC CRASH, a randomised placebo-controlled trial of intravenous corticosteroid in adults with head injury-outcomes at 6 months. Lancet 2005; 365(9475): 1957-9.
2.   Roberts I, Perel P, Prieto-Merino D, et al. Effect of tranexamic acid on mortality in patients with traumatic bleeding: prespecified analysis of data from a randomised controlled trial. Br Med J 2012; 345: e5839.
3.   Perel P, Kawahara T, Roberts I, CRASH-2 Collaborators, et al. Effect of tranexamic acid in traumatic brain injury: a nested randomised, placebo controlled trial (CRASH-2 Intracranial Bleeding Study). Br Med J 2011; 343: d3795.
4.   Dewan Y, Komolafe EO, Mejia-Mantilla JH, et al. CRASH-3 - tranexamic acid for the treatment of significant traumatic brain injury: study protocol for an international randomized, double-blind, placebo-controlled trial. Trials 2012; 13: 87.
5.   Brain Trauma Foundation, et al. Guidelines for the management of severe traumatic brain injury. J Neurotrauma 2007; 24 Suppl 1: S1-2.

24 F, T, T, F, F

Patients can present with hyperglycaemia and metabolic acidosis from a variety of causes. A diagnosis of diabetic ketoacidosis (DKA) requires the presence of ketonaemia (blood ketones of ≥3mmol/L) or significant ketonuria (>2+ on urine sticks), hyperglycaemia (BSL >11mmol/L or known diabetes mellitus) and acidaemia (serum bicarbonate <15mmol/L and/or venous pH <7.3).

There are also specific features which highlight increased severity. The presence of one or more of the following may indicate severe DKA. If the patient exhibits any of these signs they should be reviewed by a consultant physician and considered for referral to a level 2 environment.

- Blood ketones >6mmol/L.
- Bicarbonate level <5mmol/L.
- Venous/arterial pH <7.0.
- Hypokalaemia (<3.5mmol/L) on admission.
- GCS <12.
- SaO_2 <92% on air (with normal baseline respiratory function).
- Systolic BP <90mmHg.
- Pulse rate >100 or <60 bpm.
- Anion gap >16mmol/L.

Insulin therapy is delivered as a fixed rate intravenous insulin infusion (FRIII), started at a rate of 0.1 units/kg, aiming for a reduction in blood ketone concentration by 0.5mmol/L/hr, an increase in venous bicarbonate by 0.3mmol/L/hr, a reduction in capillary blood glucose by 3.0mmol/L/hr and maintenance of potassium between 4.0-5.5mmol/L. If these rates are not achieved, then the FRIII rate should be increased. Patients taking long-acting insulin preparations should continue these during the management of DKA and consideration should be made in starting these in newly presenting Type 1 patients. This helps to prevent rebound hyperglycaemia on stopping the FRIII. Oral medication may need to be suspended if oral intake is deemed an aspiration risk. Resolution of DKA is defined by a serum ketone level of <0.6mmol/L and venous pH >7.3. Urinary ketones will still be present following resolution of the metabolic picture.

1.	Savage MW, Dhatariya KK, Kilvert A, *et al*. Joint British Diabetes Societies guideline for the management of diabetic ketoacidosis. *Diabet Med* 2011; 28: 508-15.

25 F, F, F, T, F

Levosimendan is a calcium sensitiser. It increases the sensitivity of cardiac muscle to calcium without increasing the concentration of intracellular calcium ions, therefore having a positive inotropic effect. It causes vascular smooth muscle relaxation by opening ATP-sensitive potassium channels thereby reducing preload and afterload. Physiological effects include:

- Improved myocardial oxygen supply.
- Augmentation of coronary and renal blood flow.
- Reduction in systemic vascular resistance, systolic blood pressure, pulmonary capillary wedge pressure and pulmonary artery pressure.
- Reduction in coronary vascular resistance.
- Reduction in myocardial oxygen consumption.

Diastolic relaxation is not impaired by its use. Levosimendan can be used with β-blockers. The half-life of levosimendan is about 1 hour (compared with a few minutes for noradrenaline) and therefore a loading dose is required (6-24µg/kg over 10 minutes).

1. Pathak A, Lebrin M, Vaccaro A, *et al*. Pharmacology of levosimendan: inotropic, vasodilatory and cardioprotective effects. *J Clin Pharm Ther* 2013; 38(5): 341-9.
2. De Keulenaer BL. The case for levosimendan. *Crit Care Resusc* 2008; 10(3): 180.

26   F, T, T, F, T

Thrombotic thrombocytopaenia purpura (TTP) is a rare thrombotic microangiopathy, occurring due to a deficiency of a specific von Willebrand factor cleaving protein known as ADAMTS13. The condition has an untreated mortality of 90% and thus it is incumbent on all physicians potentially caring for the critically ill to identify it early and institute effective therapy.

The diagnostic pentad includes acute kidney injury, altered mental state, low platelets, fever and microangiopathic haemolytic anaemia. Not all features are necessary to make the diagnosis; up to 35% of patients present without neurological features for instance.

Platelet transfusions are essentially contraindicated in the absence of serious bleeding. Treatment options include plasmapheresis as first line, fresh frozen plasma administration, steroids, rituximab and aspirin.

1.   Scully M, Hunt BJ, Benjamin S, *et al.* Guidelines on the diagnosis and management of thrombotic thrombocytopenic purpura and other thrombotic microangiopathies. *Br J Haematol* 2012; 158(3): 323-35.

27   F, T, T, F, F

Needle decompression is the emergency treatment of a life-threatening tension pneumothorax. A 14-gauge cannula is inserted into the pleural cavity in the second intercostal space in the mid-clavicular line to allow air under tension in the pleural space to escape. The site of insertion for a chest drain is partly dictated by the position of the collection clinically, and radiologically, ultrasound can be used to guide placement. In all other cases, the drain should be sited in the 5th intercostal space, just anterior to the mid-axillary line and directed cephalad for air and caudally for fluid or blood. Paracentesis (peritoneal tap) is usually performed in the right or left iliac fossae, but in the case of tense ascites for therapeutic tap, it can be performed in the midline, 1cm below the umbilicus. Within the femoral triangle lie the femoral vein, artery and nerve; lateral to medial — femoral nerve, femoral artery, femoral vein. Therefore, a central venous catheter inserted into the femoral vein will lie medial to the femoral nerve and femoral artery. Ultrasound should be used to guide the placement of the needle for pericardiocentesis wherever possible. When this is not available a landmark technique can be employed. The point of needle insertion is immediately below and to the left of the xiphisternum, between the xiphisternum and the left costal margin.

1.   Whiteley SM, Bodenham A, Bellamy MC. *Churchill's Pocketbooks, Intensive Care*, 3rd ed. London, UK: Churchill Livingstone Elsevier, 2010.
2.   Bickle I, Hamilton P, Keppy R, McCluskey D. *Clinical Skills for Medical Students - a Hands-on Guide*, 2nd ed. Knutsford, UK: Pastest, 2005.
3.   Ellis H, Mahadevan V. *Clinical Anatomy, Applied Anatomy for Students and Junior Doctors*, 12th ed. Chichester, UK: Wiley-Blackwell, 2010.

28   T, F, T, F, F

Clostridium difficile causes 15%-25% of all cases of antibiotic-associated diarrhoea, ranging in severity from mild diarrhoea to pseudomembranous colitis which can be associated with a high mortality. Old age, recent hospital admission and immunosuppression are important risk factors. The development of diarrhoea after 72 hours of hospital admission if receiving antibiotics is a strong risk factor. Testing of stool for the presence of *C. difficile* toxin confirms the diagnosis with high sensitivity. Antibiotics associated with a high rate of *C. difficile* infection include β-lactams, cephalosporins and clindamycin. The onset of diarrhoea is commonly during or just after receiving antimicrobial therapy but may range from a few days after the initiation of treatment up to several weeks after cessation. Although stool culture has high sensitivity, the specificity is low, because the rate of asymptomatic carriage of *C. difficile* among hospitalised patients is quite high. Such carriers are often isolated depending on hospital infection control policies.

1.   Bartlett JG, Gerding DN. Clinical recognition and diagnosis of *Clostridium difficile* infection. *Clin Infect Dis* 2008; 46 (Supplement 1): S12-8.

29   F, F, F, T, F

The peak incidence of vasospasm following subarachnoid haemorrhage occurs between days 5-10. The MASH (Magnesium for Aneurysmal Subarachnoid Haemorrhage) 2 trial demonstrated no benefit to magnesium supplementation, and 'triple H' therapy is now suggested to be potentially harmful. MAP targets aim to restore cerebral perfusion pressure, with a target of >60mmHg until the aneurysm is protected (to limit the risk of further bleeding), then a target of >90mmHg following protection. These targets are mainly based on expert consensus. The ISAT (International Subarachnoid Haemorrhage Trial) study demonstrated that in patients with a ruptured intracranial aneurysm, disability-free survival at 1 year was significantly higher in patients treated with endovascular coiling compared with neurosurgical clipping. Clipping is now restricted to aneurysms that are not amenable to endovascular treatment such as those with wide necks where coiling is less effective.

1.   Dorhout Mees SM, Algra A, Vandertop WP, *et al.* Magnesium for aneurysmal subarachnoid haemorrhage (MASH-2): a randomised placebo-controlled trial. *Lancet* 2011; 380(9836): 44-9.

2. Treggiari MM, Walder B, Suter PM, Romand J. Systematic review of the prevention of delayed ischaemic neurological deficits with hypertension, hypervolaemia and haemodilution therapy following subarachnoid haemorrhage. *J Neurosurgery* 2003; 98: 978-84.
3. Molyneux A, Kerr R, Stratton I, *et al*. International Subarachnoid Aneurysm Trial (ISAT) of neurosurgical clipping versus endovascular coiling in 2143 patients with ruptured intracranial aneurysms: a randomised trial. *Lancet* 2002; 360(9342): 1267-74.

30   F, F, F, T, T

Cardiopulmonary exercise testing (CPET) is a tool used to quantify the risk of peri-operative complications. It can be used to triage patients and assess the need for postoperative critical care management. Patients use a static cycle ergometer while gas analysis, 12-lead continuous ECG, non-invasive blood pressure and oxygen saturation measurements are performed. The oxygen consumption, carbon dioxide production, respiratory exchange ratio and the anaerobic threshold are calculated. As work increases, muscle uses more oxygen and this is provided by increasing the cardiac output and increasing the oxygen extraction ratio. VO_2 increases linearly with cardiac output until a peak oxygen extraction ratio of 75% is reached. At this point oxygen demand outstrips supply and the anaerobic threshold (AT) is reached.

Patients considering undertaking major surgery should be able to perform >4 METs (metabolic equivalents), which is equivalent to climbing at least 1 flight of stairs. An AT of less than 11ml/kg/min is predictive of an increased relative risk of cardiorespiratoty morbidity and mortality following major surgery, and such patients are therefore most likely to benefit from postoperative critical care admission. Contraindications to CPET are broadly the same as those to cardiac exercise ECG stress testing, and include severe aortic stenosis, acute myocardial infarction and acutely decompensated heart failure.

1. Agnew N. Preoperative cardiopulmonary exercise testing. *Contin Educ Anaesth Crit Care Pain* 2010; 10(2): 33-7.

31 F, T, F, F, T

Counterpulsation is a term that describes balloon inflation in diastole and deflation in early systole. It is contraindicated in patients with aortic regurgitation as it worsens the magnitude of regurgitation. The intra-aortic balloon pump (IABP) catheter is inserted percutaneously into the femoral artery but other routes of access include subclavian, axillary, brachial, or iliac arteries. Helium is often used because its low density facilitates rapid transfer of gas from the console to the balloon. It is also easily absorbed into the blood stream in case of rupture of the balloon. An IABP is used for stabilisation of patients with acute myocardial infarction referred for urgent cardiac surgery. The use of IABP in this setting decreases left ventricular afterload, increases cardiac output, and increases coronary and systemic perfusion, facilitating the patient's weaning from cardiopulmonary bypass.

1.   Krishna M, Zacharowski K, Principles of intra-aortic balloon pump counter-pulsation. *Contin Educ Anaesth Crit Care Pain* 2008; 9: 24-8.

32 T, T, F, T, F

A QRS duration of >120ms is associated with an increased likelihood of seizures, while a QRS of >160ms is predictive of acute dysrhythmias. As such any prolongation should be managed aggressively. Bicarbonate is the mainstay of treatment, although current feeling suggests it may be the sodium contained that is actually advantageous and thus hypertonic saline may be of equal benefit. This has not as yet been proven in human studies.

Intralipid® has an emerging evidence base and can be considered on a case to case basis. National guidance is available as well as useful information through the TOXBASE portal (www.toxbase.org).

Normalisation of pH is best attempted through metabolic treatments rather than the ventilator, due to the additional effect of sodium on the stability of conduction channels.

Intubation and ventilation is not without risk and should be reserved for selected patients such as those with neurological deterioration requiring airway protection.

1. Body R, Bartram T, Azam F, Mackway-Jones K. Guidelines in Emergency Medicine Network (GEMNet): guideline for the management of tricyclic antidepressant overdose. *Emerg Med J* 2010; 28(4): 347-68.

33 F, T, T, F, F

The donor heart has its own sinoatrial node (but this is not innervated) which controls the graft heart rate. As there is no autonomic innervation, only drugs or manoeuvres that act directly on the heart will have an effect. Due to denervation of β-adrenergic receptors, β-adrenergic blockers have an increased antagonistic effect working on the sinoatrial and atrioventricular nodes. The Valsalva manoeuvre and carotid sinus massage will have no effect since there is no vagal innervation to the heart and thus the efferent limb of the baroreceptor reflex is lost. Coronary arteries retain their vasodilatory responsiveness to nitrates and metabolic demands. The coronaries can develop atherosclerosis, but due to denervation the patient will experience no angina pain with ischaemia or infarction. During exercise any increase in cardiac output from increased heart rate or contractility depends both on the increase in venous return and circulating catecholamines. Therefore, this response may be delayed.

1. Bersten AD, Soni N. *Oh's Intensive Care Manual*, 6th ed. Philadelphia, USA: Butterworth Heinemann, Elsevier, 2009.

34 F, F, T, T, F

The role of the precordial thump is de-emphasised and should not be attempted unless the arrest was witnessed and monitored, for example, in the cardiac catheterisation lab. Delivery of drugs via a tracheal tube is no longer recommended — if intravenous (IV) access cannot be achieved drugs should be administered by the intraosseous (IO) route. When treating ventricular fibrillation/ventricular tachycardia cardiac arrest, adrenaline 1mg is given once chest compressions have restarted after the third shock and then every 3-5 minutes (during alternate cycles of CPR). In the 2005 guidelines, adrenaline was given just before the third shock. This subtle change in the timing of adrenaline administration is to separate the timing of drug delivery from attempted defibrillation. It is hoped that this will result in more efficient shock delivery and less interruption in chest compressions. Amiodarone 300mg is also given after the third shock.

1. Resuscitation Council (UK). Advanced life support 2011. London, UK: Resuscitation Council (UK). https://www.resus.org.uk/pages/als.pdf (accessed 25th February 2015).

35 T, T, F, T, F

Therapeutic hypothermia has been trialled in the management of the post-cardiac arrest syndrome, traumatic brain injury and neonatal encephalopathy. Increased rates of bleeding, pneumonia, sepsis, hyperglycaemia and myocardial dysfunction have all been reported with its use. Benefits must be carefully weighted against risk, in light of the limited evidence base supporting practical use.

There is no evidence to suggest an independent link to worsening renal function

1. Luscombe M, Andrzejowski JC. Clinical applications of induced hypothermia. *Contin Educ Anaesth Crit Care Pain* 2006; 6(1): 23-7.
2. Nolan JP, Morley PT, Vanden Hoek IL, *et al.* Therapeutic hypothermia after cardiac arrest: an advisory statement by the advanced life support task force of the International Liaison Committee on Resuscitation. *Circulation* 2003; 108(1): 118-21.

36 T, F, F, T, F

Necrotising fasciitis (NF) is a clinical diagnosis and is the most serious presentation of necrotising soft tissue infection. Prompt recognition of NF and intervention are essential as mortality is directly proportional to time to intervention. Classification by microbial source of infection gives four subtypes. Type 1 infections are the most common form, accounting for 70-80% of cases. They are polymicrobial and wound isolates identify, on average, four different organisms. Type 2 is caused by *Streptococcus pyogenes*, with or without *Staphylococcus aureus* and account for 20-30% of cases. Type 3 is most commonly caused by *Vibrio spp*. It is uncommon but carries a high mortality. Type 4 describes fungal cases. As the infection starts at the level of the subcutaneous fat and deep fascia, in the early stages of the disease, erythema and oedema of the skin are not obvious and the extent of the infection is clinically unclear. Skin bullae, blisters, crepitus, skin fluctuation, necrosis and gangrene are seen in the later stages of the disease. Antibiotics are unable to penetrate infected necrotic tissue because of the thrombogenic nature of the process, so aggressive surgical debridement is the first priority. Empiric therapy includes a broad-spectrum agent (such as piperacillin/tazobactam or meropenem), which can be combined with clindamycin. Clindamycin is included in antibiotic therapy as it is known to switch off toxin production. If methicillin-resistant *Staphylococcus aureus* (MRSA) is suspected, linezolid is preferred to vancomycin as it inhibits exotoxin production. If Group A *Streptococcus* alone is responsible, then antibiotics can be rationalised to a combination of penicillin and clindamycin.

1.   Davoudian P, Flint NJ. Necrotizing fasciitis. *Contin Educ Anaesth Crit Care Pain* 2012; 12(5): 245-50.

37   F, F, T, F, F

Rhabdomyolysis is the dissolution of striated muscle, leading to leakage of muscle cell contents, including electrolytes, myoglobin and sarcoplasmic proteins. Increased hepatic metabolism can lead to an absence of measured myoglobinuria despite significant muscle breakdown, as myoglobin tends to peak well in advance of the creatinine kinase levels. The mainstay of treatment is aggressive resuscitation and fluid replacement aiming for a degree of haemodilution and prevention of acute kidney injury.

Alkalinisation of the urine aims to increase the solubility of the brown granular casts formed by Tamm-Horsfall protein/myoglobin complexes, to facilitate urinary drainage. Sodium bicarbonate should be titrated to a urinary pH >7. The evidence that this reduces the incidence of acute kidney injury is limited however. Hypocalcaemia is often seen in the early stages due to sequestration within damaged cells.

1.   Bosch X, Poch E, Grau JM. Rhabdomyolysis and acute kidney injury. *New Engl J Med* 2009; 361: 62-72.

38   F, F, T, T, T

A pressure ulcer is defined as an area of localised damage to the skin and underlying tissue caused by pressure, shear, friction or a combination of these. There are multiple risk assessment scales used to assess the risk of a patient developing pressure ulcers; they include the Norton, Waterlow and Braden scales. Using the NPUAP-EPUAP Pressure Ulcer Classification System, ulcers are classified into four grades: Grade I have non-blanchable erythema of intact skin; Grade II are partial-thickness skin loss involving the epidermis, dermis or both — the ulcer is superficial and presents clinically as an abrasion or blister; Grade III have full-thickness skin loss with damage that may extend down to underlying fascia; Grade IV have extensive destruction or damage to muscle, bone or supporting structures with or without full-thickness skin loss. Risk factors for the development of pressure ulcers are exaggerated in critically ill patients. As many of the risk factors are considered in severity of illness scores, it follows that the APACHE II score highly correlates with the occurrence of pressure ulcers. Current guidance suggests that patients should be repositioned at least every 6 hours to decrease the risk of developing pressure ulcers. In the critically ill, due to the higher risks, patients should be repositioned every 2-3 hours if their clinical condition allows.

1.   Keller BPJA, Wille J, van Ramshort B, van der Werken C. Pressure ulcers in intensive care patients: a review of risks and prevention. *Intensive Care Med* 2012; 28: 1379-88.
2.   National Institute for Health and Care Excellence. Pressure ulcer management. The prevention and management of pressure ulcers in primary and secondary care. NICE clinical guideline 179. London, UK: NICE, 2014. www.nice.org.uk (accessed 25th February 2015).

39   F, T, F, T, T

At therapeutic doses, paracetamol is mainly metabolised by conjugation to inactive metabolites. A reactive metabolite, N-acetyl-p-benzoquinoneimine (NAPQI), is formed by the process of oxidation. When paracetamol is ingested in large amounts, more NAPQI is formed, sulphation conjugation pathways are saturated, and NAPQI binds covalently to sulfhydryl (SH-) groups. These groups normally can be provided by glutathione, but when hepatic glutathione stores are depleted, NAPQI binds to cellular proteins and causes hepatic cell injury.

Glutathione depletion may occur in patients for a variety of reasons thus increasing the risk of liver injury following overdose of paracetamol. These include malnutrition, alcoholism and the use of a variety of hepatic enzyme-inducing drugs including many antiepileptics, rifampicin, efavirenz, nevirapine, and St John's Wort.

1. Hinson JA, Roberts DW, James LP. Mechanisms of acetaminophen-induced liver necrosis. *Handb Exp Pharmacol* 2010; 196: 369-405.
2. Ferner RE, Dear JW. Management of paracetamol poisoning. *Br Med J* 2011; 342: d2218.

40 F, F, T, F, F

Tumour lysis syndrome (TLS) is a potentially life-threatening complication of massive cellular lysis in cancer, often encountered in bulky, rapidly progressive or chemo-sensitive tumours. It is most commonly seen in haematological malignancy. Hypocalcaemia is a hallmark feature due to precipitation of ionised calcium with phosphate, which is released in large quantities in tumour lysis. Other laboratory features of TLS include: increase in serum uric acid by >25% from baseline; increase in serum potassium by >25% from baseline; increase in serum phosphate by >25% from baseline.

Drugs acting to prevent the formation of uric acid (allopurinol), or increase the formation of allantoin from uric acid (rasburicase), have a key role in treatment. Steroids are of no demonstrable benefit.

Intravenous hydration and rasburicase are first-line treatments and prophylaxis agents in high-risk groups. Rasburicase is a synthetic urate oxidase enzyme and breaks down uric acid which, along with the presence of hyperphosphataemia, is a principal cause of acute kidney injury in TLS-associated renal failure.

Paper 1 Answers

1.   Tosi P, Barosi G, Lazzaro C, *et al.* Consensus conference on the management of tumor lysis syndrome. *Haematologica* 2008; 93(12): 1877-85.

41 T, F, T, F, F

Submassive PE is defined as acute pulmonary embolism (PE) without systemic hypotension (defined as systolic BP <90mmHg), but with evidence of right ventricular dysfunction or myocardial necrosis. Evidence of right ventricular dysfunction might include a dilated right ventricle on CT or echo imaging, new right bundle branch block, or elevated B-natriuretic peptide >90pmol/ml. Evidence of myocardial necrosis would be suggested by troponin elevated above the reference range. The management of submassive PE presents a therapeutic challenge; although there are data to suggest a modest mortality benefit from thrombolysis, there is also a significant risk of intracranial haemorrhage. The most recent European Society of Cardiology guidelines do not recommend thrombolysis for submassive (intermediate risk) pulmonary embolism in the absence of haemodynamic decompensation.

1.   Jaff MR, McMurtry MS, Archer SL, *et al.* Management of massive and submassive pulmonary embolism, iliofemoral deep vein thrombosis, and chronic thromboembolic pulmonary hypertension. *Circulation* 2011; 123: 1788-830.
2.   Konstantinides SV, Torbicki A, Agnelli G, *et al.* 2014 ESC guidelines on the diagnosis and management of acute pulmonary embolism. *Eur Heart J* 2014; 35: 3033-80.

42 F, F, F, F, T

Clinical examination must be carried out by two physicians working together and must be repeated. In UK practice, at least one of the doctors must be a consultant and both must have been fully registered with the GMC for more than 5 years. Neither must be potentially involved in the care of patients who may be in receipt of organs donated by the patient to be tested.

A summary of the tests to be undertaken are as follows:

- The pupils are fixed and do not respond to sharp changes in light intensity (mesencephalon, II and III) — dilatation not necessarily present.
- There is no corneal reflex (pons, V and VII).
- The oculo-vestibular reflexes are absent (pons, VIII, III, IV, VI).
- No motor responses within the cranial nerve distribution in response to stimulation of any somatic area.
- There is no cough reflex response to bronchial stimulation by a suction catheter placed down the trachea to the carina, or gag response to stimulation of the posterior pharynx with a spatula (medulla, IX, X).
- There is no evidence of spontaneous respiration or respiratory effort during the apnoea test.

Spinal reflexes to a sternal rub can still occur and do not signify brainstem function. Measurement of visual evoked responses is not required for confirmation of brainstem death.

1. Academy of Medical Royal Colleges. A code of practice for the diagnosis and confirmation of death, October 2008. http://www.aomrc.org.uk/aomrc/admin/reports/_docs/DofD-final.pdf (accessed 23rd July 2014).

43 T, T, T, F, F

Pulse oximeters employ only two wavelengths of light and, therefore, can distinguish only two main substances, haemoglobin (Hb) and oxyhacmoglobin (O_2Hb). When carboxyhemoglobin (COHb) and methaemoglobin (MetHb) are also present, four wavelengths are required to determine the 'fractional SaO_2': i.e. (O_2Hb × 100)/(Hb + O_2Hb + COHb + MetHb).

In the presence of elevated COHb levels, oximetry tends to over-estimate the true oxygen saturation by the quantity of COHb present. Elevated MetHb levels also may cause inaccurate oximetry readings and will often give a falsely low saturation. Anaemia does not appear to affect the accuracy of pulse oximetry. Even severe hyperbilirubinemia does not affect the accuracy of pulse oximetry. Intravenous dyes such as methylene blue and indocyanine green can cause falsely low readings. Nail polish, if blue, green or black, causes inaccurate SpO_2 readings, whereas acrylic nails do not interfere with pulse oximetry readings. Vasoconstriction may reduce pulsatile flow of blood at the extremities, which is required for accurate determination of SpO_2.

1.   Jubran A. Pulse oximetry. *Crit Care* 1999; 3(2): R11-7.

44   F, T, F, T, T

Treatment strategies in thrombotic thrombocytopaenia purpura (TTP) are limited. Plasma exchange (PEX) is the mainstay of therapy and has reduced mortality when commenced early in the condition from 90% to 10-20%. The British Society of Haematology has recently produced a stepwise treatment algorithm focused around the use of PEX. Additional treatments listed include solvent/detergent-treated fresh frozen plasma, packed red cells and high-dose steroid therapy.

Platelet transfusions are contraindicated regardless of count, unless there is life-threatening bleeding.

In addition, with neurological or cardiac involvement, rituximab is recommended. When the platelet count increases to above 50 x 10^9/L, aspirin and the consideration of low-molecular-weight heparin (LMWH) are also recommended.

1.   Scully M, Hunt BJ, Benjamin S, *et al*. Guidelines on the diagnosis and management of thrombotic thrombocytopenic purpura and other thrombotic microangiopathies. *Br J Haematol* 2012; 158(3): 323-35.

45   T, T, T, T, F

Once a diagnosis of brainstem death is made, the patient is legally dead and the focus of management moves away from a patient-focused approach to an organ management approach; therefore, insertion of new invasive monitoring (if indicated) is often considered appropriate. In the potential heart-beating donor, the patient is still alive and management is guided by the principle of 'best interest'. The patient's best interests require reference to all factors affecting the person's interests. Guidance from the Department of Health states that "delaying the withdrawal of treatment may be considered to be in the best interests of someone who wanted to be a donor if this facilitates donation and does not cause the person harm or distress, or place them at significant risk of experiencing harm or distress". The Human Tissue Act 2004 recognises that the wish to donate may have been recorded or stated in various ways — verbally, by having a Donor Card, in writing or via the NHS Organ Donor Register (ODR), all of which are regarded as equally valid forms of consent. The family have no authority at law to overturn the known wishes of an individual. However, if the wishes of the individual are not known then the authority of decision making passes to the nominated representative and then to the family. There is no age restriction for self-registration on the ODR. Children under the age of 12 years at the time of registration are assumed to have been registered by their parents, while those of 12 years and over are assumed to have self-registered.

1. Gordon JK, McKinlay J. Physiological changes after brain stem death and the management of the heart-beating donor. *Contin Educ Anaesth Crit Care Pain* 2012; 12(5): 225-9.
2. Murphy P, Adams J. Ethicolegal aspects of organ donation. *Contin Educ Anaesth Crit Care Pain* 2013; 13(4): 125-30.

46   T, F, T, F, F

As most drugs, fluids and equipment are given/used on a weight basis, it is important to determine a child's weight as soon as possible. If weighing the child is impractical, weight can be estimated using the formulae outlined in Table 1.1.

Table 1.1. Calculation of ideal body weight in children.	
0-12 months	Weight (kg) = (0.5 x age in months) + 4
1-5 years	Weight (kg) = (2 x age in years) + 8
6-12 years	Weight (kg) = (3 x age in years) + 7

Both cuffed and uncuffed tubes are suitable for an infant or child undergoing emergency intubation. The size of an uncuffed endotracheal tube can be estimated using various formulae including:

Internal diameter (mm) = (Age/4) + 4
Length for an oral tube (cm) = (Age/2) + 12

Although the presenting rhythm for most paediatric arrests is non-shockable, should the child have a shockable rhythm, 4J/kg is the energy selection of the asynchronous DC shock. In a cardiac arrest situation, the dose of adrenaline is 10µg/kg, administered either intravenously or intraosseously. Five minutes after a seizure has started, a benzodiazepine should be administered. If intravenous access is secured this is intravenous lorazepam 100µg/kg, if not, buccal midazolam (0.5mg/kg) or rectal diazepam (0.5mg/kg) should be given. If a child presents in shock with bradycardia and vagal activity is suspected, 20µg/kg atropine should be administered.

1.   Samuels M, Wieteska S. Advanced Life Support Group. *Advanced Paediatric Life Support. The Practical Approach*, 5th ed. Oxford, UK: Wiley-Blackwell, 2005.

47   T, T, F, T, T

The Wells score (Table 1.2) is a validated tool to guide management in venous thromboembolism.

Those with Wells scores of two or more have a 28% chance of having deep vein thrombosis (DVT); those with a lower score have 6% odds.

Table 1.2. Wells score or criteria: (possible score -2 to 9).

1.	Active cancer (treatment within last 6 months or palliative)	+1 point
2.	Calf swelling ≥3cm compared to asymptomatic calf (measured 10cm below tibial tuberosity)	+1 point
3.	Swollen unilateral superficial veins (non-varicose, in symptomatic leg)	+1 point
4.	Unilateral pitting oedema (in symptomatic leg)	+1 point
5.	Previous documented DVT	+1 point
6.	Swelling of entire leg	+1 point
7.	Localised tenderness along the deep venous system	+1 point
8.	Paralysis, paresis or recent cast immobilisation of lower extremities	+1 point
9.	Recently bedridden ≥3 days, or major surgery requiring regional or general anaesthetic in the past 12 weeks	+1 point
10.	Alternative diagnosis at least as likely	-2 points

A V/Q can be used if the chest X-ray is normal, and is therefore a useful investigation in many patients, although in the ICU population the chest X-ray is rarely normal. Otherwise a CT pulmonary angiogram (CTPA) is more sensitive and specific in such cases and is considered the gold standard for diagnosis. Seventy percent of proven cases of PE have proximal DVTs. In active cancer cases with a proven pulmonary embolism, lifelong anticoagulation may be required. The evidence base suggests that treatment with low-molecular-weight heparin is superior to treatment with a vitamin K antagonist (e.g. warfarin) in the first 6 months, although the preferred anticoagulant beyond this period is not clear. The reported incidence of venous thromboembolism in critically ill patients varies in the literature but is between 20 and 60% varying by patient group (trauma and stroke very high incidence).

1. National Institute for Health and Care Excellence. Venous thromboembolic diseases. NICE clinical guideline 144. London, UK: NICE, 2012. www.nice.org.uk (accessed 25th February 2015).

48 T, F, F, T, F

Iron overdose is often fatal and requires aggressive early management. Tablets are radiopaque and thus in the case of polypharmacy overdose or reluctant disclosure, a chest and abdominal X-ray can confirm ingestion.

Iron does not bind to activated charcoal and so administration is futile. Transition through the gastric tract and bloodstream absorption can be delayed, however, and as such early presentation can sometimes be managed by mechanical means. At present, the National Poisons Information Service (NPIS) recommends the consideration of whole bowel irrigation as a primary means of reducing tablet absorption rather than direct endoscopic retrieval.

Chelation therapy is recommended for all those with symptoms of severe toxicity, regardless of serum iron level. Following an initial phase of severe gastroenteritis, patients with a significant ingestion may develop metabolic acidosis, cardiovascular instability, central nervous system symptoms such as coma, and hepatic dysfunction. In other patients, treatment with desferrioxamine should be delayed pending serum iron level measurements at 4-6 hours. A level of 90µmol/L should prompt consideration of treatment, as should a deterioration in clinical state or a lower level rising on serial assay. Caution is due to the side effects of desferrioxamine, which include hypotension, ARDS and thrombocytopaenia. Proton pump inhibitors are not a feature of most treatment guidelines, although in general, medications that increase stomach pH reduce the absorption of iron.

1.   Savitt DL, Hawkins HH, Roberts JR. The radiopacity of ingested medications. *Ann Emerg Med* 1987; 16(3): 331-9.
2.   http://www.toxbase.org/Poisons-Index-A-Z/I-Products/Iron/#ironwithin6 (accessed 28th August 2014).
3.   Howland MA. Risks of parenteral deferoxamine for acute iron poisoning. *J Toxicol Clin Toxicol* 1996; 34: 491-7.

49 T, T, F, F, F

A systematic review and meta-analyses have shown that 'high-intensity' units (staffed by intensivists as opposed to intensive care consultation only on request) have lower case-adjusted mortality. Consensus opinion suggests that a maximum ratio of one fully trained intensivist to 14 patients is acceptable, although this will depend on casemix. Non-clinical inter-hospital transfer has been shown to lengthen critical care stay but not to increase mortality. Patients admitted over the weekend have a 10% increase in odds ratio of death compared with those admitted in the week, possibly due to lower staffing levels and less experienced providers of care. There is no randomised controlled trial of night-time discharges from intensive care, but retrospective cohort studies suggest an excess mortality for patients discharged between 2100 and 0700 compared with daytime discharges.

1. Wilcox ME, Chong CA, Niven DJ. Do intensivist staffing patterns influence hospital mortality following ICU admission? A systematic review and meta-analyses. *Crit Care Med* 2013; 41(10): 2253-74.
2. Ward NS, Afessa B, Kleinpell R, *et al.* Intensivist/patient ratios in closed ICUs: a statement from the Society of Critical Care Medicine Taskforce on ICU Staffing. *Crit Care Med* 2013; 41(2): 638-45.
3. Barratt H, Harrison DA, Rowan KM, Raine R. Effect of non-clinical inter-hospital critical care unit to unit transfer of critically ill patients: a propensity-matched cohort analysis. *Crit Care* 2012; 16(5): R179.
4. Aylin P, Yunus A, Bottle A, *et al.* Weekend mortality for emergency admissions. A large, multicentre study. *Qual Saf Health Care* 2010; 19(3): 213-7.
5. Priestap FA, Martin CM. Impact of intensive care unit discharge time on patient outcome. *Crit Care Med* 2006; 34(12): 2946-51.

50 F, T, F, T, F

The CURB-65 score is a validated clinical prediction tool used to determine mortality related to community-acquired pneumonia. It is recommended by the British Thoracic Society. There is one point for each risk factor with a maximum score of 5:

* **C**onfusion of new onset (defined as an Abbreviated Mental Test score of 8 or less).
* **U**rea greater than 7mmol/L.

- **R**espiratory rate of 30 breaths per minute or greater.
- **B**lood pressure less than 90mmHg systolic or diastolic blood pressure 60mmHg or less.
- Age **65** or older.

It predicts the risk of death at 30 days. This increases as the score increases. The score is used as a method to evaluate where the patient may be able to be managed:

- 0-1: treat as an outpatient.
- 2-3: consider hospital admission or watch very closely as an outpatient.
- 4-5: requires hospitalisation with consideration of intensive care admission.

Polymerase chain reaction (PCR) analysis of respiratory tract samples is the method of choice for the diagnosis of mycoplasma pneumonia. Urinary legionella antigen is the method of choice for the diagnosis of legionella pneumonia. Patients with high-severity pneumonia should be treated with parenteral antibiotics as soon as the diagnosis is made. Community-acquired pneumonia may be complicated by a parapneumonic effusion or empyema signified by a pH <7.2; this should be drained early. Steroids are not a recommended treatment except in cases of exacerbation of chronic obstructive pulmonary disease (COPD).

1.   British Thoracic Society. Guideline for the management of community-acquired pneumonia in adults. Update 2009. https://www.brit-thoracic.org.uk/guidelines-and-quality-standards/community-acquired-pneumonia-in-adults-guideline (accessed 30th September 2014).

51   T, F, F, F, T

The previous American and European Consensus Conference definition of ARDS was updated to the modern Berlin definition in 2012. This new definition addressed several suggested failings of the previous; namely issues of reliability and validity relating to limited clarity of timeframe/onset, interpretation of chest radiograph criteria and issues with identifying hydrostatic oedema.

The new definition incorporates four specific aspects to diagnosis. These aspects focus specifically on timing of onset, supporting chest imaging, the origin of pulmonary oedema and oxygenation.

When calculating P/F gradient the new definition mandates positive end-expiratory pressure (PEEP) or continuous positive airway pressure (CPAP) of at least 5cmH$_2$O. The Murray score is a grading system for severity of ARDS and plays a limited role in initial diagnosis. Respiratory failure must be unexplained by cardiac failure/fluid overload in the new definition, but specific pulmonary artery occlusion pressure measurements are discounted in light of the move away from PA catheter placement in recent years. pH plays no role and acute precipitant is now a specific diagnostic aspect as above. Additional advantages to the new diagnosis include more robust diagnostic criteria for inclusion in research studies and the added value of clearly defining hypoxia despite PEEP.

Paper 1 Answers

1. Bernard GR, Artigas A, Brigham KL, *et al.* The American-European Consensus Conference on ARDS: definitions, mechanisms, relevant outcomes, and clinical trial coordination. *Am J Respir Crit Care Med* 1994; 149(3 pt 1): 818-24.
2. The ARDS definition taskforce. Acute respiratory distress syndrome, the Berlin definition. *JAMA* 2012; 307(23): 2526-33.
3. Murray JF, Matthay MA, Luce JM, Flick MR. An expanded definition of the adult respiratory distress syndrome. *Am Rev Respir Dis* 1988; 138: 720-3.

52 T, F, T, F, F

Concerning the initial assessment and resuscitation of an upper GI bleed, platelets should not be offered to those who are not actively bleeding and are stable. For those who are bleeding, a platelet count of less than 50 x 10^9/L should be used as a threshold for transfusion. FFP should be given if the INR is greater than 1.5 times normal. The NICE guidelines reserve recombinant factor VIIa for the management of bleeding where all other methods have failed.

1. National Institute for Health and Care Excellence (NICE). Acute upper gastrointestinal bleeding: management. NICE clinical guideline 141. London, UK: NICE, June 2012. www.nice.org.uk (accessed 25th February 2015).

53 T, F, F, T, F

The Brain Trauma Foundation (BTF) guidelines provide level 1 to 3 graded recommendations on the early aspects of management for TBI. They aim for consensus, evidence-based recommendations to encourage best practice.

Prehospital triage direct to neurosciences centres is recommended both within the BTF guidelines and the recent NICE head injury guidelines. Therapeutic hypothermia for refractory intracranial hypertension is currently a therapy of equipoise and the subject of a randomised controlled trial. As such it cannot be recommended based on current evidence. Hyperventilation can cause cerebral vasoconstriction leading to poor blood supply to the ischaemic penumbra and as such is not recommended routinely. Osmotherapy with hypertonic saline should ideally be instituted in the presence of ICP monitoring, but BTF guidelines support use in the deteriorating patient with no additional explanation for compromise, or the patient with clinical signs of impending transtentorial herniation. Routine monitoring of intracranial pressure is not necessarily recommended in the presence of a normal CT brain scan.

1. https://www.braintrauma.org/coma-guidelines/searchable-guidelines (accessed 26th February 2015).
2. Badjatia N, Carney N, Crocco TJ, et al. Guidelines for prehospital management of traumatic brain injury 2nd edition. Prehosp Emerg Care 2008; 12 Suppl 1: S1-52.
3. Hodgkinson S, Pollit V, Sharpin C, Lecky F, for the Guideline Development Group. Early management of head injury: summary of updated NICE guidance. Br Med J 2014; 348: g104.
4. http://www.eurotherm3235trial.eu/home/index.phtml (accessed 26th February 2015).
5. Bullock MR, Povlishok JT. Brain Trauma Foundation; American Association of Neurological Surgeons; Guidelines for the management of severe traumatic brain injury. J Neurotrauma 2007; 24 Suppl 1: S1-106.

54 F, F, F, T, T

Generic scoring systems can be divided into: those that assess disease severity on admission and use it to predict outcome, such as the Acute Physiology and Chronic Health Evaluation (APACHE), Simplified Acute Physiology Score (SAPS), and Mortality Probability Model (MPM); scores that assess the presence and severity of organ dysfunction, such as the

Multiple Organ Dysfunction Score (MODS), Sequential Organ Failure Assessment (SOFA); and scores that assess nursing workload use, such as the Therapeutic Intervention Scoring System (TISS). Outcome prediction scores are used to provide an indication of the risk of death of groups of ICU patients; they cannot, however, provide individual prognostication. The APACHE II score is the world's most widely used severity of illness score. There are 12 physiological variables and the effects of age and chronic health status are incorporated directly into the model, weighted according to their relative impact, to give a single score with a maximum of 71. The variables for the APACHE II score were selected and weighted by a panel of experts. For the APACHE III score they were selected by multiple logistic regression analysis. The SAPS includes 20 variables related to patient characteristics prior to admission, the circumstances of admission and physiological derangement 1 hour before and 1 hour after ICU admission. SAPS 3 can be customised to predict hospital mortality in seven geographical regions. The SOFA (Sequential Organ Failure Assessment) looks at 6 organs and scores the function of each with possible scores of 0-24. A score of >15 correlates with a mortality rate of 90% and it has been shown that an increase in SOFA score during the first 48 hours in the ICU, independent of the initial score, predicted a mortality of at least 50%, while a decrease was associated with an ICU mortality rate of just 27%.

1.   Vincent JL, Moreno R. Clinical review: scoring systems in the critically ill. *Crit Care* 2010; 14: 207.

55   F, F, T, T, F

Encephalitis is inflammation of the brain. When associated with meningitis it is named meningoencephalitis. It is often associated with a high morbidity and mortality. Symptoms include headache, fever, confusion, drowsiness, and fatigue. More advanced and serious symptoms include seizures or convulsions, tremors and hallucinations.

Viral encephalitis can occur either as a direct effect of an acute infection, or as one of the sequelae of a latent infection. The most common causes of acute viral encephalitis are *Herpes simplex* (Types 1 and 2), poliovirus, measles virus, and JC virus. Other potential causes include bacterial, rickettsial and certain parasitic or protozoal infestations, such as toxoplasmosis, malaria, or primary amoebic meningoencephalitis. These organisms more often cause encephalitis in people with compromised immune systems. Lyme disease may also cause encephalitis. *Cryptococcus neoformans* is a cause of fungal encephalitis in the immunocompromised. *Streptococci*, *Staphylococci* and certain Gram-negative bacilli cause cerebritis prior to the formation of a brain abscess. CT scans are often normal although temporal lobe changes may be seen, and MRI scans offer greater sensitivity. However, a CT scan is useful in ruling out other causes of an altered sensorium that might require different management (for example, subdural haematoma). In patients with *Herpes simplex* encephalitis, an electroencephalograph may show sharp waves in one or both of the temporal lobes.

Many types of viral encephalitis may be treated with specific anti-viral treatments or immunomodulatory medications such as steroids or intravenous immunoglobulin. However, even with specific therapies, certain types of encephalitis have mortality rates of between 10-30%. *Herpes simplex* virus encephalitis (HSE) has a mortality rate of up to 30% with specific anti-viral treatment, and 70-80% without the treatment.

1. HPA England. Encephalitis. www.hpa.org.uk (accessed 26th February 2015).
2. Rozenberg F, Deback C, Agut H. *Herpes simplex* encephalitis: from virus to therapy. *Infectious Disorders Drug Targets* 2011; 11(3): 235-50.
3. Dowell E. Death from encephalitis (acute stage). Factsheet. Updated 2011. http//www.encephalitis.info (accessed 13th July 2014).

56 F, F, F, F, T

The concept of care bundles and marginal gains has received a lot of attention in critical care. There are several bundle mnemonics to encourage attention to detail when applying basic intensive care for the critically ill, but Jean-Louis Vincent's publication of the FAST-HUG concept is one of the best known and remains pioneering.

FAST-HUG recommends strict attention to the following daily aspects of critical care: feeding; analgaesia; sedation; thromboembolic prophylaxis;

head of the bed elevation; stress ulcer prevention; glucose control. There has been a recent suggestion that this daily bundle should be increased to FAST HUGS BID, in an effort to factor in spontaneous breathing trials, bowel care, indwelling catheter removal and de-escalation of antibiotics.

1.   Vincent JL. Give your patient a fast hug (at least) once a day. *Crit Care Med* 2005; 33(6): 1225-9.
2.   Vincent JL, Hatton KW. Critically ill patients need "FAST HUGS BID" (an updated mnemonic). *Crit Care Med* 2009; 37(7): 2326-7.

57   F, F, F, F, T

Duty of confidentiality continues after the patient dies. Personal information can be disclosed in specific circumstances but the next of kin has no rights to access the patient's records. Genetic information about a patient might, at the same time, also be information about others with whom the patient shares genetic links. If the patient refuses consent to disclose information which may benefit others (help them get prophylaxis or other preventative treatments or interventions), there is a balance between the need to respect patient confidentiality and the duty to protect others from serious harm. In certain circumstances the duty to others may override the duty to the patient and the information can be legally disclosed. The next of kin is not able to authorise disclosure of confidential information about a patient, whether the patient is dead or alive, unless they have been authorised to make decisions on behalf of, or if they are appointed to support and represent, a mentally incapacitated patient.

The Caldicott Committee (chaired by Dame Fiona Caldicott) produced a report on the review of patient-identifiable information in 1997. They identified six key principles: justify the purpose of using confidential information; do not use patient-identifiable information unless absolutely necessary; use the minimum necessary patient-identifiable information that is required; access to patient-identifiable information should be on a strict need-to-know basis; everyone with access to patient-identifiable information should be aware of their responsibilities; understand and comply with the law.

Caldicott Guardians are senior people in the NHS, local authority social care, and partner organisations, who are responsible for protecting the confidentiality of patient information and enabling appropriate information sharing. They advise on confidentiality issues but do not make decisions about a patient's medical care. By law, each NHS institution must employ a Caldicott Guardian.

1. Department of Health. Confidentiality, NHS Code of Practice. London, UK: Department of Health, 2003.
2. NHS Executive. Health Service Circular. Caldicott Guardians. HSC 1999/012. London, UK: NHS Executive, 1999.
3. Department of Health. The Caldicott Committee - Report on the review of patient-identifiable information. London, UK: Department of Health, 1997.
4. General Medical Council. Confidentiality, guidance for doctors. London, UK: General Medical Council, 2009.

58   T, T, T, F, F

Risk factors for aneurysmal subarachnoid haemorrhage (SAH) include hypertension, smoking, alcohol abuse, and use of sympathomimetic drugs such as cocaine. In addition to female sex, the risk is increased if there is a history of previous aneurysmal SAH (with or without a residual untreated aneurysm) and a strong family history and certain genetic syndromes, such as autosomal dominant polycystic kidney disease and collagen disorders such as Type IV Ehlers-Danlos syndrome. The size at which aneurysms rupture appears to be smaller in those patients with the combination of hypertension and smoking than in those with either risk factor alone. There does not appear to be an increased risk of aneurysmal SAH in pregnancy, delivery, and puerperium.

1. AHA/ASA Guideline. Guidelines for the management of aneurysmal subarachnoid haemorrhage. A guideline for healthcare professionals from the American Heart Association/American Stroke Association. Stroke 2012; 43: 1711-37.

59   T, F, F, T, F

Ventilator-associated pneumonia (VAP) is the most common hospital-acquired infection in patients receiving mechanical ventilation, with a considerable morbidity burden. The diagnosis is challenging. Both the Clinical Pulmonary Infection Score (CPIS) and Hospital in Europe Link for Infection Control through Surveillance (HELICS) scoring systems have been developed as decision tools, but are limited in their sensitivity and specificity.

A VAP is defined as a hospital-acquired pneumonia occurring after 48 hours of mechanical ventilation. There has been justifiable criticism of this definition and the current trend appears to be moving in favour of a tiered approach, recognising various ventilator-associated events as a ventilator-associated condition (VAC), an infection-related ventilator-associated condition (IVAC) and probable/possible VAP.

Ventilator care bundles include a series of measures attempting to reduce the incidence of VAP. These measures often include tapered high-volume low-pressure cuffs, head elevation, subglottic suction, mouthcare and occasionally selective oral and digestive tract decontamination. Of all these, subglottic suction appears to have the best evidence base for reduction in events. Early VAP is usually caused by oropharyngeal flora, including streptococcal and staphylococcal organisms. Late VAP is usually a result of infection by Gram-negative enteric organisms.

1. Hunter JD. Ventilator-associated pneumonia. *Br Med J* 2012; 344: e3325.
2. Zilberberg MD, Shorr AF. Ventilator-associated pneumonia: the clinical pulmonary infection score as a surrogate for diagnostics and outcome. *Clin Infect Dis* 2010; 51(S1): S131-5.
3. Raoof S, Baumann MH. Ventilator-associated events: the new definition. *Am J Crit Care* 2014; 23(1): 7-9.
4. Muscedere J, Rewa O, McKechnie K, *et al*. Subglottic secretion drainage for the prevention of ventilator-associated pneumonia: a systematic review and meta-analysis. *Crit Care Med* 2011; 39(8): 1985-91.

60 T, T, F, F, F

There are four basic ethical principles in healthcare — respect for autonomy, beneficence, non-maleficence and justice. Autonomy is 'deliberate self rule'; if we have autonomy we can make our own decisions on the basis of deliberation. Respect for autonomy is the moral obligation to respect the autonomy of others in so far as such respect is compatible with equal respect for the autonomy of all potentially affected. Beneficence and non-maleficence can be thought of together and the aim is to produce net benefit over harm — beneficence with non-maleficence. In the case of blood and bone marrow donation, autonomy retains primacy over non-maleficence. Justice is the moral obligation to act on the basis of fair adjudication between competing claims. Explicit consent is consent which is expressed orally or in writing. Implied consent is that which can be inferred if the patient has been informed that information is to be disclosed, the purpose and extent of the disclosure, and that they have a right to object, but have not objected.

The exchange of information between doctor and patient is central to informed consent; however, if a patient does not wish to know the details about their condition or treatment, this should be respected as far as possible. When a procedure is contemplated for a patient lacking capacity, the treating medical professional can authorise this if it is deemed in the patient's best interests. While it is good practice to obtain assent from the patient's next of kin this is not a legal requirement.

1.   Gillon R. Medical ethics: four principles plus attention to scope. *Br Med J* 1994; 309: 184
2.   General Medical Council. Consent: patients and doctors making decisions together. London, UK: GMC, 2008.

61 D

The main concern in this patient is potentially Guillain-Barré syndrome and more specifically the Miller Fisher variant. A pressing concern is to assess the need for ventilatory support secondary to respiratory muscle weakness. Urgent spirometry should be organised to measure forced vital capacity. If this is less than 1L, he may need intubation and invasive ventilation and needs to be monitored in a high-care area where such intervention is immediately available. He will need a cardiac monitor and ECG due to potential autonomic dysfunction related to the condition. Stool cultures should be taken to rule out the *Campylobacter jejuni* organism. He will need a lumbar puncture and if CSF analysis demonstrates a raised protein level, then discussions with a local neurology centre for immunoglobulin therapy should be undertaken. Occasionally, MRI scans of brain and spinal cord may be needed but is not a first-line investigation. Nerve conduction studies may also be performed.

1.   Richards KJC, Cohen AT. Guillain-Barré syndrome. *Br J Anaesth CEPD Rev* 2003; 3(2): 46-9.

62 B

Catabolism in critical illness means that patients can rapidly develop an energy deficit when critically unwell. Often, a recovery state will mean that oral feeding is inadequate and so great care should be placed on the provision of adequate nutrition. This is always individually patient orientated.

High gastric volumes should prompt consideration of prokinetic therapy, but the duration is usually less than 5 days and in most centres will be limited to 24-48 hours as per best evidence. Propofol contains 1kcal/ml of energy and as such ongoing use should be factored into calculation of all feeds, enteral or parenteral. MUST is a screening tool based on knowledge of the patient's body mass index, acute illness status and evidence of recent weight loss, and patients scoring highly should have a more detailed assessment.

The EPaNIC (Early versus late Parenteral Nutrition In Critically ill patients) trial showed a reduction in mortality with late commencement of parenteral nutrition (PN) in this patient cohort, thus leading to the prevailing practice of late PN in patients unable to meet calorific requirements. In the largest randomised controlled trial to date, glutamine and antioxidant supplementation led to an increased mortality in patients with critical illness undergoing mechanical ventilation.

1.   Grant K, Thomas R. Prokinetic drugs in the intensive care unit: reviewing the evidence. *J Intensive Care Soc* 2009; 10(1): 34-7.
2.   Casaer MP, Mesotten D, Hermans G, *et al*. Early versus late parenteral nutrition in critically ill adults. *New Engl J Med* 2011; 365: 506-17.
3.   Heyland D, Muscedere J, Wischmeyer PE, *et al*. A randomized trial of glutamine and antioxidants in critically ill patients. *New Engl J Med* 2013; 368: 1489-97.

63 E

This patient has taken a significant amount of paracetamol with a delayed presentation to hospital. Despite correct initial management she has developed liver failure. There is no indication for renal replacement therapy or bicarbonate at this stage. The INR should be monitored to assess progression of her liver failure; FFP is not required unless there is active bleeding or surgical intervention is planned. Vitamin K should, however, be administered to ensure that vitamin K deficiency is not the cause of her coagulopathy. She does not meet the criteria for the super-urgent liver transplant scheme post-paracetamol poisoning but as she is clinically deteriorating her case should be discussed with a liver unit.

Criteria for placement on the super-urgent liver transplant scheme are outlined in Table 1.3.

Table 1.3. Criteria for placement on the super-urgent liver transplant scheme.

1. pH <7.25 more than 24 hours after overdose and after fluid resuscitation
2. Coexisting prothrombin time >100 seconds or INR >6.5, and serum creatinine >300µmol/L or anuria, and grade 3-4 encephalopathy
3. Serum lactate more than 24 hours after overdose >3.5mmol/L on admission or >3.0mmol/L after fluid resuscitation
4. Two of the criteria from no. 2 with clinical evidence of deterioration

1.   National Health Service Blood and Transplant, Liver Advisory Group. POL 195/2. Liver transplantation: selection criteria and recipient registration. London, UK: NHSBT, 2014.

64 A

Generous IV crystalloid should be administered. Active warming is important but intravenous fluid resuscitation should be the first priority — if the patient is actively rewarmed without correcting volume status this is likely to precipitate vasodilatation and significant hypotension. Mannitol and furosemide may be used to try and improve renal perfusion (with limited evidence base) but is not initial treatment. His potassium is above the normal range and may need renal replacement therapy if it does not correct with adequate fluid resuscitation, but the patient does not need urgent haemodialysis.

1. Lerma EV, Berns JS, Nissenson SR. In: *Current Diagnosis and Treatment, Nephrology and Hypertension.* McGraw-Hill Companies, 2009: 109-12.

65 D

Hepatorenal syndrome is defined as a functional renal failure in patients with liver disease and portal hypertension. It can be segregated into Type 1, caused by splanchnic vasodilatation and a reduction in cardiac output leading to profound renal vasoconstriction, or Type 2, where slow incipient renal failure leads to progressive accumulation of refractory ascites. It is essentially a diagnosis of exclusion following assessment for the multiple other causes of renal failure in the critically ill patient with cirrhosis. International consensus diagnostic criteria are available.

Treatment is focused on improving renal blood flow via intravascular volume repletion and vasoconstriction. Albumin is the preferred choice for volume repletion in these patients, but usually commenced at a higher loading dose of 1g/kg up to 100g/day. Terlipressin is likely to be the most efficacious agent, due to splanchnic vasoconstriction and redirection of central blood flow to vital organs. There has been much study of terlipressin in this context, including case reports, prospective cohort data and randomised controlled trials. A Cochrane review is supportive and the majority of consensus guidelines recommend the agent as first-line alongside volume resuscitation.

Transjugular intrahepatic portosystemic shunt (TIPSS) has a role but is a therapy with limited supporting evidence. Furosemide infusion is likely to exacerbate the situation. Dopamine is an unlikely choice for cardiac output support following recent trial data to suggest a higher rate of adverse events over noradrenaline infusion.

1. Lata J. Hepatorenal syndrome. *World J Gastroenterol* 2012; 18(36): 4978-84.

2.   Salerno F, Gerbes A, Ginès P, *et al.* Diagnosis, prevention and treatment of hepatorenal syndrome in cirrhosis. *Gut* 2007; 56(9): 1310-8.
3.   Gluud LL, Christensen K, Christensen E, Krag A. Terlipressin for hepatorenal syndrome. *Cochrane Database Syst Rev* 2012; 9: CD005162.
4.   De Backer D, Biston P, Devriendt J, *et al.* Comparison of dopamine and norepinephrine in the treatment of shock. *N Engl J Med* 2010; 362: 779-89.

66   C

The poor clinical grade of this woman's subarachnoid haemorrhage (SAH) puts her at higher risk of complications, especially within the first 72 hours. The Lindegaard ratio is the ratio of flow velocity in the ipsilateral middle cerebral and internal carotid arteries; a ratio of >3 is suggestive of vasospasm. Whilst she is hyponatraemic, a serum sodium level of 130 does not usually cause such profound symptomatology. A rebleed would be seen as high-attenuating areas within the subarachnoid space. Normally the temporal horns of the lateral ventricles are not visible on CT; a cresenteric appearance is suggestive of hydrocephalus. Clinical seizures are uncommon, occurring in only 1-7% of patients. Had the CT not shown a cause for her deterioration, an EEG should be performed to exclude a non-convulsive status epilepticus.

1.   Luoma A, Reddy U. Acute management of aneurysmal subarachnoid haemorrhage. *Contin Educ Anaesth Crit Care Pain* 2013; 13(2): 52-8.

67   A

Acute liver failure (ALF) is a syndrome defined by the occurrence of encephalopathy, coagulopathy and jaundice in an individual with a previously normal liver. In the UK, the most common cause is paracetamol overdose.

Cerebral oedema occurs in up to 80% of cases of ALF and a high index of suspicion is required if the Glasgow Coma Scale deteriorates. The development of cerebral oedema reflects impaired cellular osmoregulation in the brain. This is thought to be due to an excess of glutamine which in turn is a consequence of high ammonia levels.

ALF is commonly associated with renal failure of an oliguric nature. Significant paracetamol overdose can be associated with renal dysfunction due to a combination of acute tubular necrosis and pre-renal failure secondary to decreased renal blood flow. The existence of renal dysfunction in ALF carries a poor prognosis and may be associated with increased mortality. Significant uraemia sufficient to cause a decreased conscious level would be unlikely to have developed in the timeframe given in the question.

In this scenario given the fact that there is no mention of pre-existing chronic liver disease, the most likely cause of the neurological deterioration is cerebral oedema.

1.   Wai KL, Murphy N. Management of acute liver failure. *Contin Educ Anaesth Crit Care Pain* 2004; 4(2): 40-3.

 68   A

This patient has an incomplete spinal cord injury, suggestive of a motor level at approximately C5/6 but with preservation of sensation below the level of that lesion. The American Spinal Injury Association (ASIA) international standards for neurological classification of spinal cord injury is the preferred tool for classification, ranging from A (complete motor and sensory) through B (sensory incomplete), C (motor incomplete with MRC <3), D (motor incomplete with MRC >2) and E (normal). Medical Research Council (MRC) grading scale refers to an assessment of an individual muscle group regarding strength with or without the interference of gravity.

The need for an accurate initial classification reflects the importance of prognosis and ongoing tailored rehabilitation in this patient cohort. In addition, it can allow for early detection of injury progression or resolution of spinal shock.

1.   Marino RJ, Barros T, Biering-Sorensen F, *et al*. International standards for neurological classification of spinal cord injury. *J Spinal Cord Med* 2003; 26(suppl 1): S50-6.
2.   Paternostro-Sluga T, Grim-Stieger M, Posch M, *et al*. Reliability and validity of the Medical Research Council (MRC) scale. *J Rehabil Med* 2008; 40(8): 665-71.

 B

The Berlin definition (2013) of ARDS no longer differentiates between ARDS and acute lung injury (ALI). ARDS is categorised as being mild (PaO_2/FiO_2 26.6-39.9kPa), moderate (PaO_2/FiO_2 13.3-26.6kPa) or severe (<13.3kPa). The definition has four key components (Table 1.4).

Table 1.4. The Berlin definition of ARDS.

1.	Acute — onset over 1 week or less
2.	Bilateral opacities consistent with pulmonary oedema on CXR or CT
3.	PaO_2/FiO_2 <300mmHg (40kPa) with a minimum PEEP of 5cm H_2O
4.	Not fully explained by cardiac failure or fluid overload

Transfusion-related acute lung injury is defined as new-onset acute lung injury that occurs during or within 6 hours of transfusion, not explained by another acute lung injury risk factor. Ventilator-associated pneumonia is, by definition, only diagnosed after the patient has been ventilated for more than 48 hours. The good cardiac function as demonstrated by echocardiography suggests that cardiogenic pulmonary oedema is unlikely and the stroke volume variation of 14% (assuming full mechanical ventilation) suggests that the patient is still fluid-responsive.

1.   ARDS Definition Task Force, Ranieri VM, Rubenfeld GD, Thompson BT, *et al*. Acute respiratory distress syndrome: the Berlin Definition. *JAMA* 2012; 307(23): 2526-33.
2.   Toy P, Lowell C. TRALI - definition, mechanisms, incidence and clinical relevance. *Best Pract Res Clin Anaesthesiol* 2007; 21(2): 183-93.

70 D

As per the British Thoracic Society (BTS) guidance in 2011, asthmatics with acute severe signs as this patient, nebulised bronchodilator therapy should be used as first line. Steroids may follow and can be either intravenous or orally administered. Intravenous magnesium should be given to patients with acute severe asthma not responding to initial therapy or with life-threatening features. Antibiotics are not always warranted in such cases. A chest X-ray will be required urgently to exclude other causes of shortness of breath, but this should not delay the administration of nebulised bronchodilators.

1. British guideline on the management of asthma: a national clinical guideline 101. BTS/SIGN, May 2011.

71 A

Acute traumatic spinal cord injury (SCI) can lead to devastating clinical consequences. SCI can be divided into the primary injury and secondary cord damage as a result of hypotension/hypoxia and ongoing mechanical instability. In keeping with traumatic brain injury, the majority of clinical care is currently focused on aggressive early intervention to prevent secondary injury.

In high cervical cord lesions, the interruption of sympathetic outflow can lead to the development of neurogenic shock, with resultant bradycardia and hypotension. This is often confused with spinal shock, which actually refers to the absence of reflexes below the level of the lesion caused by a transient 'concussion' of the cord.

In hypotension, haemorrhage should be actively excluded prior to the assumption of neurogenic shock. In order to prevent secondary injury, a MAP of 90mmHg is currently recommended by expert consensus to optimise perfusion and reduce the ischaemic penumbra. Abdominal breathing reflects failure of the thoracic musculature to facilitate work of breathing and is often an impending sign of the need for respiratory support.

1.   http://www.lifeinthefastlane.com/trauma-tribulation-016 (accessed 11th July 2014).
2.   Casha S, Christie S. A systematic review of intensive cardiopulmonary management after spinal cord injury. *J Neurotrauma* 2011; 28: 1479-95.

72   A

Delirium is an independent predictor of increased mortality at 6 months and longer length of stay in ventilated intensive care patients. The Confusion Assessment Method for the ICU (CAM-ICU) and the Intensive Care Delirium Screening Checklist (ICDSC) are the most valid and reliable delirium monitoring tools in adult ICU patients. Three subtypes of delirium have been characterised: hyperactive, hypoactive and mixed. There are many predisposing factors for the development of delirium, including severe infection and patient-ventilator dyssynchrony. Treatment of delirium includes pharmacological and non-pharmacological measures. For the management of hyperactive or mixed delirium, haloperidol is the treatment of choice; however, it carries a risk of QT prolongation and should not be used if the QTc is prolonged (>450ms). Benzodiazepines should be used to manage specific delirium syndromes such as alcohol withdrawal and otherwise avoided as they can contribute to the delirium. Midazolam or propofol could be used as rescue therapy for rapid tranquillisation if other therapy is failing and the patient poses a danger to themselves or attending staff, but should otherwise be avoided. There is increasing evidence that atypical antipsychotics, such as quetiapine, may reduce the duration of delirium in adult ICU patients, but there are no parenteral formulations and they are therefore not suitable in this case due to the patient's ileus. In mechanically ventilated adult ICU patients at risk of developing delirium, dexmedetomidine infusions administered for sedation may be associated with a lower prevalence of delirium compared with benzodiazepine infusions, and are recommended in these patients. As an α1-agonist, dexmedetomidine will have an antihypertensive effect which may also help in this case.

1.   The Intensive Care Society. Detection, prevention and treatment of delirium in critically ill patients. London, UK: ICS, 2006.
2.   Barr J, Fraser GL, Puntillo K, *et al*. Clinical practice guidelines for the management of pain, agitation, and delirium in adult patients in the intensive care unit. *Crit Care Med* 2013; 41: 263-306.

Paper 1 Answers

73 D

This case points towards myasthenia gravis (MG). MG affects 1 in 10,000 of the population predominantly towards younger woman (20-30-year-old) and older males (60-70-year-old). This is indicated by the weakness worsened on fatigability. Multiple sclerosis may well present as a relapsing/remitting disease or rapidly progressive depending on its presentation. Dermatomyositis is a form of a connective tissue disease which classically presents with proximal weakness and a purple coloured rash over the eyelids (heliotrope) and Gottron's papules (thickened and discoloured skin over the knuckles of both hands). Creatinine kinase may be elevated in dermatomyositis. GBS affects individuals of all ages, although there is a bimodal tendency towards young adults and the elderly. The majority of cases of GBS occur within a month of either a respiratory or gastrointestinal infection. There is usually back pain followed by an ascending neuropathy and autonomic symptoms. Sub-acute degeneration of the spinal cord is associated with degeneration of the posterior and lateral columns of the spinal cord as a result of vitamin B12 deficiency. Patients present with weakness of legs, arms, trunk, tingling and numbness that progressively worsens. Vision changes and change of mental state may also be present. Bilateral spastic paresis may develop and pressure, vibration and touch sense are diminished.

1.   Marsh S, Ross N, Pittard A. Neuromuscular disorders and anaesthesia. Part 2: specific neuromuscular disorders. *Contin Educ Anaesth Crit Care Pain* 2011; 11(4): 115-8.

74 C

Panton-Valentine leukocidin (PVL) is one of several extracellular toxins produced by *Staphylococcus aureus*, which can be either methicillin-sensitive or methicillin-resistant. Although usually associated with skin and soft tissue infections, it can result in necrotising haemorrhagic pneumonia. Early identification and aggressive antimicrobial therapy is key, although diagnosis can be challenging. A rise in incidence has led to developing interest from a critical care perspective. The mortality rate can be as high as 75% in these cases.

The Health Protection Agency have produced guidelines on the diagnosis, investigation and management of this challenging infective condition. The presence of necrotic tissue raises the concern that the use of flucloxacillin will result in concentrations just above the minimum inhibitory concentration (MIC) and as such, use may increase the production of PVL *in vivo*. In addition, vancomycin is not recommended due to poor extracellular fluid levels and penetration of lung tissue. There is little evidence to support the benefit of nebulised pentamidine.

The consensus recommendation is for empirical combination therapy with clindamycin, linezolid (for toxin clearance) and rifampicin (for intracellular clearance of staphylococci). In addition, the use of 2g/kg intravenous immunoglobulin should be strongly considered as adjunctive care, for its ability to neutralise exotoxins and superantigens. This dose can be repeated at 48 hours if there is a failure to respond.

1. McGrath B, Rutledge F, Broadfield E. Necrotising pneumonia, *Staphylococcus aureus* and Panton-Valentine leukocidin. *J Intensive Care Soc* 2008; 9(2): 170-2.
2. http://www.hpa.org.uk/webc/hpawebfile/hpaweb_c/1204186171881 (accessed 19th September 2014).

75 D

Fluid responsiveness is defined as the ability of the heart to increase its stroke volume significantly in response to volume expansion because of the presence of biventricular preload reserve. Static markers of preload include central venous pressure, pulmonary artery occlusion pressure and cardiac chamber dimensions; however, they fail to predict volume responsiveness reliably at anything but the lowest and highest ranges.

Dynamic markers include heart-lung interaction indexes and passive leg raising. Heart-lung interaction indexes are validated in patients receiving full mechanical ventilation. Insufflation may decrease right ventricular filling through a decrease in venous return. This leads to a decrease in right ventricular stroke volume and thus, 2-3 beats later, usually during expiration, a decrease in left ventricular stroke volume. Thus, cyclical changes in left ventricular stroke volume occur in cases of biventricular preload reserve. The magnitude of the cyclical changes correlate with the degree of fluid responsiveness. Respiratory variation of arterial pulse pressure, peak Doppler aortic blood velocity, descending aorta blood velocity (or blood flow) and pulse contour-derived stroke volume variation are all examples of heart-lung interaction indexes. However, they cannot be used in patients who are spontaneously breathing or are receiving tidal volumes <7ml/kg or in patients with arrhythmias. Passive leg raising (PLR) — lifting the legs by 45° from the horizontal position induces a gravitational transfer of blood from the lower limbs and increases preload. A real-time cardiac output monitor is used to detect an increase in cardiac output. In patients with spontaneous breathing activity and/or cardiac arrhythmias, a PLR-induced increase (>10%) in descending aorta blood flow (oespophageal Doppler) or a PLR-induced increase (>12.5%) in pulsed Doppler stroke volume (echocardiography) can accurately detect fluid responsiveness.

1.   Waldmann C, Soni N, Rhodes A. *Oxford Desk Reference Critical Care*. Oxford, UK: Oxford University Press, 2008.

76   B

BTS guidance suggests in patients with pre-existing chest disease and greater than 50 years, a pneumothorax should be treated as secondary. If they are breathless and/or have a pneumothorax greater than 2cm, then this should be treated with a chest drain. If the pneumothorax is small (1-2cm), then this could be aspirated with a 16G or 18G cannula. If successful, then the patient should be observed for 24 hours. If unsuccessful, then this should be followed by chest drain insertion. If the pneumothorax is less than 1cm on admission then they should be observed with high-flow oxygen unless oxygen-sensitive.

1.   British Thoracic Society: pneumothorax guidelines 2010. *Thorax* 2010; 65 (Suppl II): 18-31.

77 A

A blocked tracheostomy requires a timely response and stepwise intervention. Whilst all the above options are reasonable, the lack of movement in the Mapleson C circuit and absent capnograph trace implies near complete obstruction. The most important next step is to focus on identification of whether this is due to distal tracheobronchial occlusion or misplacement of the tracheostomy itself.

To this end, the National Tracheostomy Safety Project algorithim suggests the passage of a suction catheter as the first step to discriminate. If this passes freely, then aspiration of a sputum plug may resolve the issue. Although bronchoscopy would be equally reasonable, the urgency in this situation would render set up and use inappropriate.

Following an inability to pass a suction catheter, deflating the cuff is the final step in an attempt to render the tracheostomy patent. If this achieves no benefit, the tracheostomy should be removed and the patient oxygenated via the mouth with an occluded stoma, or via the mouth and stoma prior to attempts at resiting a definitive airway. This could be via oral endotracheal intubation (with the tube sited distal to the stoma) or intubation of the stoma itself.

1.   http://www.tracheostomy.org.uk/Resources/Printed%20Resources/Patent%20 Airway%20Algorithm.pdf (accessed 16th June 2014).

78 A

This patient is in cardiogenic shock and he has signs of end-organ hypoperfusion. An assessment of his fluid status must be made and treatment instigated as appropriate. Once fluid status is optimised, an inodilator, such as milrinone would be an appropriate treatment of choice. Milrinone is a selective phosphodiesterase 3 inhibitor in cardiac myocytes and vascular smooth muscle. It increases cardiac contractility, vasodilates and improves diastolic relaxation, thus reducing preload, afterload and systemic vascular resistance. Dobutamine is a synthetic catecholamine with a strong affinity for β-1 and β-2 receptors. It is also an inodilator but often causes a tachycardia and is therefore inappropriate in this case. At low doses, cardiac contractility is improved without greatly affecting peripheral resistance but vasoconstriction dominates at higher infusion rates. Noradrenaline is a potent α-1 agonist with modest β agonist activity. It mainly increases systolic, diastolic and pulse pressure and has minimal effect on cardiac output. Adrenaline has high affinity for β-1, β-2 and α-1 receptors in cardiac and smooth muscle, causing positive inotropy and chronotropy and an increase in systemic vascular resistance. Digoxin has some positive inotropic effect but has no place in the management of the low cardiac output state seen in this case.

1.   Overgaard CB, Dzavik V. Inotropes and vasopressors: review of physiology and clinical use in cardiovascular disease. *Circulation* 2008; 118: 1047-56.

79   C

If the timing of onset can be defined then urgent thrombolysis is indicated within a 4.5-hour period. The last time this patient was seen well was at 2200 and the onset of symptoms could have occurred anytime between then and when he was found. Trials are ongoing to determine whether thrombolysis can be safely given in patients who wake up with symptoms of a stroke in whom time of onset cannot be determined. As an intra-cerebral bleed has been excluded he should receive 300mg aspirin for 14 days followed by 75mg clopidogrel. Blood pressure should not be reduced acutely in the first 24-48 hours. Criteria for acute blood pressure reduction include: hypertensive encephalopathy, hypertensive nephropathy, hypertensive cardiac failure/myocardial infarction, pre-eclampsia/eclampsia, aortic dissection and intracerebral bleed with systolic BP greater than 200mmHg. Consideration should be given to blood pressure reduction to less than 185/110mmHg or lower in people who are candidates for thrombolysis.

1.   National Institute for Health and Care Excellence. Stroke: diagnosis and initial management of acute stroke and transient ischaemic attack. NICE clinical guideline 68. London, UK: NICE, 2008. www.nice.org.uk (accessed 25th February 2015).

80   D

Malignant cerebral artery syndrome carries a mortality of 80%. This is often due to increasing cerebral oedema refractory to medical treatment, leading to eventual herniation and death. Rising intracranial pressure as a result of stroke is theoretically amenable to surgical intervention, in the same way as traumatic brain injury. There has been much study of this in the last decade.

Three trials form the base of the evidence, appraised together in a systematic review in the *Lancet Neurology* and more recently, a meta-analysis by the Cochrane group. Patients included age up to 60 in the earlier trials, and with the recent publication of DESTINY 2 (DEcompressive Surgery for the Treatment of malignant INfarction of the middle cerebral arterY), there is clear consensus that equipoise remains in the elderly and there may well be a role for surgery. The role of decompression in stroke is at present restricted to malignant middle artery syndromes, and the timing of intervention has ranged up to 96 hours in clinical trials.

The modifided Rankin Scale (mRS) is often used to assess outcome as a measure of disability. This ranges from 0 (best) to 5 (worst) and 6 as death. Most systematic reviews report mortality as a primary outcome, which is often improved with the intervention. However, there has been no trial proving a clear improvement in the proportion of survivors with moderate or less disability (mRS <or equal to 3). As such the intervention is currently reducing mortality but increasing the proportion of survivors with moderately severe or worse disability. As such, its use remains contentious.

1.   Vahedi K, Hofmeijer J, Juettler E, *et al.* Early decompressive surgery in malignant infarction of the middle cerebral artery: a pooled analysis of three randomised controlled trials. *Lancet Neurol* 2007; 6(3): 215-22.
2.   Cruz-Flores S, Berge E, Whittle IR. Surgical decompression for cerebral oedema in acute ischaemic stroke. *Cochrane Database Syst Rev* 2012; 1: CD003435.
3.   Jüttler E, Unterberg A, Woitzik J, *et al.* Hemicraniectomy in older patients with extensive middle-cerebral-artery stroke. *New Engl J Med* 2014; 370: 1091-100.

81 C

It is generally accepted that sedation strategies using non-benzodiazepine sedatives may be preferred over sedation with benzodiazepines to improve clinical outcomes in mechanically ventilated adult ICU patients; therefore, although midazolam may be added to a sedative regime if control is not achieved with non-benzodiazepine sedatives, it would not be the first-line sedative agent of choice. Fentanyl is metabolised in the liver to inactive metabolites and the parent drug will therefore accumulate in liver failure. Remifentanil is metabolised by non-specific plasma and tissue esterases and therefore will not accumulate in renal or hepatic failure. Dexmedetomidine is a potent α2-agonist and its use as a sedative in intensive care is increasing; there is supporting evidence of its potential to decrease the duration of mechanical ventilation and allow earlier extubation. The use of dexmedetomidine is limited by its side effects of hypotension and bradycardia, and it would therefore not be a good choice for a patient with a low blood pressure requiring a noradrenaline infusion. Thiopentone is only administered as an infusion for the management of refractory status epilepticus and a bolus can be given for the management of raised intracranial pressure (ICP). This patient's ICP lies within the normal range and therefore a bolus of thiopentone is not indicated. Causes for this patient's agitation on waking must be assessed. Alcohol withdrawal should be excluded and delirium recognised. Boluses of neuroleptic agents, benzodiazepines, α2-agonists and atypical antipsychotics should be considered, in addition to the sedative regime if delirium is diagnosed.

1.   Barr J, Fraser GL, Puntillo K, *et al*. Clinical practice guidelines for the management of pain, agitation, and delirium in adult patients in the intensive care unit. *Crit Care Med* 2013; 41(1): 263-306.
2.   Rowe K, Fletcher S. Sedation in the intensive care unit. *Contin Educ Anaesth Crit Care Pain* 2008; 8(2): 50-5.
3.   Ahmed S, Murugan R. Dexmedetomidine use in the ICU: are we there yet? *Crit Care* 2013; 17: 230.

82 B

The likelihood here is this man has had an alcohol withdrawal fit. He is at risk of further seizures if his blood sugar is not corrected. However, such patients are at risk of Wernicke's encephalopathy and giving them glucose before intravenous thiamine and other vitamins (Pabrinex®) may increase the risk of seizures related to Wernicke's encephalopathy. If glucose is given, such as in hypoglycaemic alcoholics, thiamine must be given concurrently. If this is not done, the glucose will rapidly consume the remaining thiamine reserves, exacerbating this condition. If he fits again then intravenous benzodiazepines such as lorazepam should be given.

Wernicke's encephalopathy refers to the presence of neurological symptoms caused by biochemical lesions of the central nervous system after exhaustion of B-vitamin reserves, in particular, thiamine. The condition is part of a larger group of diseases related to vitamin B1 insufficiency, including beriberi in all its forms, and Korsakoff syndrome. When Wernicke's encephalopathy occurs simultaneously with Korsakoff syndrome it is known as Wernicke-Korsakoff syndrome.

Typically, Wernicke's encephalopathy is characterised by the triad of ophthalmoplegia, ataxia, and confusion. While it is commonly observed in malnourished people with alcohol misuse, a variety of diseases can lead to Wernicke's encephalopathy such as pancreatitis, liver dysfunction, hyperemesis gravidarum, starvation and fasting.

1.   Schuckit MA. Alcohol-use disorders. *Lancet* 2009; 373(9662): 492-501.
2.   National Institute for Health and Care Excellence. Alcohol-use disorders: diagnosis and clinical management of alcohol-related physical complications. NICE clinical guideline 100. London, UK: NICE, June 2010. www.nice.org.uk (accessed 25th February 2015).
3.   Sechi G, Serra A. Wernicke's encephalopathy: new clinical settings and recent advances in diagnosis and management. *Lancet Neurol* 2007; 6(5): 442-55.

83 A

The management of intracranial hypertension is fast becoming a staple of critical care. It can be seen with both medical (hepatic failure/meningitis) and surgical (traumatic brain injury) emergencies. Failure to recognise and promptly treat can result in severe disability and ultimately death.

Recognition is based primarily on clinical findings, often supported by radiology in the sedated patient. Monitoring is mandatory if cerebral perfusion pressure is to be optimised, often requiring cardiovascular supervision/support and placement of a device to directly monitor intracranial pressure. Once this device is *in situ*, the management can be tailored to maintain intracranial pressure below a predefined threshold (often 20mmHg) using a gradient of escalating therapies.

Management is often tiered. Initial care involves the optimisation of venous drainage and cerebral perfusion pressure, through adequate sedation, supported blood pressure and good gas exchange. Following this, escalating ICP requires additional interventions, many of which lack supporting evidence. Although most data are post hoc, resuscitation with albumin is suggested to lead to worse outcomes in traumatic brain injury. Risk factors for infection following insertion of a ventriculostomy principally include duration, CSF leakage at the site, or open skull fracture. Hyperosmolar therapy is supported by level II evidence and as such is the most likely beneficial option here. Hypertonic 3% saline decreases blood viscoscity and this rheologic effect is thought to be the principal mechanism of action. Surgical decompression is usually reserved for those patients resistant to all medical management.

An excellent review article summarising these points is available.

1.   Stoccheti N, Maas AIR. Traumatic intracranial hypertension. *New Engl J Med* 2014; 370: 2121-30.

84 A

Thromboelastography (TEG®) provides information on all phases of coagulation and due to the quick turnaround time can be used to reduce inappropriate transfusion. It should be noted that the majority of the evidence base supporting the use of TEG® comes from cardiac surgery, although it is increasingly being used in trauma, vascular and bleeding critical care patients. The principle of thromboelastography is that whole blood from the patient is added to activators and placed into a cup. A pin is immersed into the blood and the cup is rotated. As the blood clots the rotational movement of the cup is transmitted to the pin. A transducer converts the torsion on the pin into a thromboelastograph. The R-time, (reaction time) for whole blood is 4-8 minutes, this is the time until initiation of fibrin formation (a 2mm amplitude on the tracing). This reflects the concentration of soluble clotting factors in the plasma. The K-time for whole blood is 1-4 minutes; this is the time period for the amplitude of the tracing to increase from 2 to 20mm. The angle (whole blood 47-74°) is the angle between a tangent to the tracing at 2mm amplitude and the horizontal midline. The K-time and the angle measure clot kinetics and the rapidity of fibrin build-up and cross-linking. The maximum amplitude (MA, whole blood 55-73mm) is the greatest vertical width achieved by the tracing and reflects the number and function of platelets and fibrinogen concentration. Clot lysis at 30 minutes (% reduction in amplitude 30 minutes after MA) and at 60 minutes show clot stability and fibrinolysis. When the decrease after maximal amplitude over 60 minutes is >15% of maximal amplitude, hyperfibrinolysis is suspected. The R-time is prolonged in this patient which suggests a deficiency in clotting factors and FFP should be administered.

1. Srivastava A, Kelleher A. Point-of-care coagulation testing. *Contin Educ Anaesth Crit Care Pain* 2013; 13(1): 12-6.
2. Bolliger D, Seeberger MD, Tanaka KA. Principles and practice of thromboelastography in clinical coagulation management and transfusion practice. *Transfus Med Rev* 2012; 26(1): 1-13.

85 B

This scenario points towards cardiogenic pulmonary oedema possibly secondary to a non-ST elevation myocardial infarction (NSTEMI). If STEMI was evident on ECG he would need stabilisation before consideration of transfer to a PCI centre. Thrombolysis would only be considered if he was too unstable to transfer, in the context of STEMI. CPAP may help as a short-term measure and may help avoid intubation and ventilation. CPAP reduces preload and causes reduction of the left ventricular transmural pressure gradient producing benefits in cardiogenic pulmonary oedema. The 3CPO (Three interventions in Cardiogenic Pulmonary Oedema) trial recruited 1069 patients with acute cardiogenic pulmonary oedema and subsequently demonstrated that non-invasive ventilation induces a more rapid improvement in respiratory distress and metabolic disturbance than did standard oxygen therapy. Unfortunately no effect was seen on short-term mortality. If this patient develops cardiogenic shock, an intra-aortic balloon pump may be indicated to augment cardiac performance and reduce myocardial oxygen consumption, although the evidence base for this is weak.

1. Gray A, Goodacre S, Newby D. Efficacy of non-invasive ventilation in patients with acute cardiogenic pulmonary oedema: the 3CPO trial. *N Engl J Med* 2008; 359: 142-51.

86 B

The primary goals of IABP counterpulsation include the reduction in myocardial oxygen demand and afterload alongside an increase in myocardial oxygen delivery and cardiac output. This is achieved through a variety of complex physiological effects secondary to increased diastolic pressure following inflation of the balloon, then deflation during systole. A review article is available.

Although previous guidance recognised the IABP as a viable option in cardiogenic shock complicating acute STEMI, appraisal of the supporting evidence has led to a rethink. A recent randomised controlled trial found no benefit of use in a prospective cohort of 600 patients. There appears to be little support in evidence, although use as a rescue measure based on expert consensus continues.

Renal blood flow should increase by up to 25%, following the increase in cardiac output. A drop in urine output raises the concern of balloon placement in a juxta-renal position.

1. Krishna M, Zachaerowski K. Principles of intra-aortic balloon counterpulsation. *Contin Educ Anaesth Crit Care Pain* 2009; 9(1): 24 8.
2. Sjauw KD, Engström AE, Vis MM, *et al*. A systematic review and meta-analysis of intra-aortic balloon pump therapy in ST-elevation myocardial infarction: should we change the guidelines? *Eur Heart J* 2009; 30(4): 459-68.
3. Thiele H, Zeymer U, Neumann FJ, *et al*. Intraaortic balloon support for myocardial infarction with cardiogenic shock. *New Engl J Med* 2012; 367: 1287-96.

87 C

Ventilator-associated pneumonia (VAP) is pneumonia in a patient who has been intubated for at least 48 hours. If a VAP is suspected every effort must be made to exclude other sources of infection. There is a lack of consensus 'gold standard' definition to test the diagnostic accuracy of potential criteria; therefore, there are multiple potential criteria to diagnose VAP, including microbiological and clinical, which lack sensitivity and specificity. The Clinical Pulmonary Infection Score (CPIS) is a diagnostic scoring 0-12, based on six variables: body temperature; leucocyte count; volume and character of tracheal secretions; arterial oxygenation; chest radiograph findings, and results of microbiological analysis. A CPIS >6 is a reasonable indicator of the presence or absence of pulmonary infection, as signified by bacterial culture. Using the CPIS this patient has a score of 7 and VAP can be diagnosed. Sputum samples should be sent in an attempt to identify a causative organism. While she also meets the criteria for acute respiratory distress syndrome (new bilateral infiltrates and an FiO_2/PaO_2 34kPa), the increase in temperature and leucocyte count suggest infection is the more likely diagnosis. Loss of the right hemi-diaphragm suggests there is a pulmonary effusion present, in this case, likely parapneumonic.

1.   Stewart NI, Cuthbertson BH. The problems diagnosing ventilator-associated pneumonia. *J Intensive Care Soc* 2009; 10(4): 266-72.
2.   Zilberberg MD, Shorr AF. Ventilator-associated pneumonia: the clinical pulmonary infection score as a surrogate for diagnostics and outcome. *Clin Infect Dis* 2010; 51(S1): S131-5.

88 A

The gross ascites is a sign of decompensation of alcohol-related liver disease. This is primarily related to sodium and water retention due to secondary hyperaldosteronism. The abdominal distension may splint the diaphragm and impair ventilation. Draining the ascites would facilitate extubation. Consensus guidelines suggest that a large-volume paracentesis should be performed in a single session with volume expansion being given once paracentesis is complete, ensuring that albumin is given (8g albumin per litre of ascites removed, equivalent to roughly 100ml of 20% albumin per 3L ascites)(level of evidence Ib; recommendation: A). This prevents cardiovascular decompensation due to fluid shifts post-drainage. Many patients with decompensated liver disease requiring intubation have a very poor prognosis, but intubation to facilitate the management of variceal bleeding carries a good short-term survival, and palliation in this situation with the information given would not be appropriate.

1.   EASL clinical practice guidelines on the management of ascites, spontaneous bacterial peritonitis, and hepato-renal syndrome in cirrhosis. *J Hepatol* 2010; 53: 397-417.
2.   Moore KP, Aithal GP. Guidelines for the management of ascites in cirrhosis. *Gut* 2006; 55 (Suppl VI): vi1-12.

89   C

The H1N1 strain of influenza A (swine flu) was responsible for a pandemic infection in 2009. Much data were collected at this time in order to assess the at-risk population and, in particular, to gauge the impact on critical care in preparation for future pandemic infections.

The most susceptible groups according to these data appeared to be infants, those with multiple respiratory comorbidities, those with a BMI >35 and women in the latter stages of pregnancy. The last two groups formed the bulk of critical care admissions. In addition, the elderly appeared to be relatively spared with the bulk of clinically relevant infection occurring in those younger than 65. This was thought to be a result of previous exposure to similar antigens and cross-reactivity. Thus, mortality rates are not linked to advancing age.

In the most recent systematic review, prophylaxis studies appear to demonstrate a reduction in the rate of symptomatic influenza both for individuals by 55% (3.05%, 95% CI 1.83-3.88%; number needed to benefit 33, 95% CI 26-55) and households. Unfortunately, treatment studies have shown little evidence of a significant mortality benefit and at best a short reduction in duration of illness.

1. The ANZIC influenza investgators. Critical care services and 2009 H1N1 influenza in Australia and New Zealand. *N Engl J Med* 2009; 361: 1925-34.
2. Jefferson T, Jones M, Doshi P, *et al.* Oseltamivir for influenza in adults and children: systematic review of clinical study reports and summary of regulatory comments *Br Med J* 2014; 348: g2545.

90 D

Intravenous drug users who inject into the bloodstream are prone to right-sided infective endocarditis typically involving the tricuspid valve, and most often caused by *Staphylococcus aureus*.

Common causative bacteria are *Staphylococcus aureus* followed by *Streptococcus viridans*. Other *Streptococci* and *Enterococci* are common causes, the latter occurring as a result of gastrointestinal or genitourinary tract abnormalities. Occasionally, a 'culture-negative' endocarditis may be due to a HACEK group of bacteria which are part of the normal dental and oropharyngeal flora (*Haemophilus*, *Actinobacillus*, *Cardiobacterium*, *Eikenella*, *Kingella*) or fungal infection. Other culture-negative causes include infections with *Coxiella* and *Chlamydia psittaci*; these are seen less frequently. *Streptococcus bovis* is commonly associated with colon cancer.

1. Mitchell RS, Kumar V, Robbins SL, *et al. Robbins Basic Pathology*, 8th ed. Saunders/Elsevier, 2007: 406-8.
2. Mathew J, Addai T, Anand A, *et al.* Clinical features, site of involvement, bacteriologic findings, and outcome of infective endocarditis in intravenous drug users. *Arch Intern Med* 1995; 155(15): 1641-8.

Paper 2
Questions

Multiple True False (MTF) questions — select true or false for each of the five stems.

1 The following are considered risk factors for intensive care unit-acquired weakness (ICUAW):

a. Hypoglycaemia.
b. Male gender.
c. Alcohol excess.
d. Severe sepsis.
e. Prolonged mechanical ventilation.

2 With regard to scoring systems in critical care:

a. There are two versions of the Acute Physiology and Chronic Health Evaluation (APACHE) score currently in use.
b. Disease-specific scoring systems include the 4T assessment tool, Blatchford score and the Wells clinical prediction rules.
c. The Sequential Organ Failure Assessment (SOFA) score can be used as a sequential indicator of organ dysfunction.
d. The AIS, ISS, and RTS are all scores designed to assess and categorise the acute trauma patient.
e. The Richmond Agitation Severity Scale (RASS) is graded as a 5-point scale.

3 A multicentre, randomised, double-blind, controlled trial is designed to compare a new antihypertensive with a placebo for the lowering of blood pressure. The null hypothesis is that there will be no difference between the measured blood pressure at the beginning of the trial and that measured at 30 days. After 30 days of treatment the blood pressure is remeasured. Statistical tests using confidence intervals of 95% deliver a p value of 0.06.

a. This is a phase 2 study.
b. Provided the trial is of good quality, the quality of evidence produced would be classified as level Ib using the GRADE system of classification.
c. A power calculation should be performed during the analysis of the data to assess the degree of change.
d. Parametric statistical tests are likely to be appropriate when analysing data from this study.
e. The null hypothesis can be rejected.

4 With regards to the use of vasopressin in patients with septic shock:

a. Vasopressin is synthesised in the posterior pituitary.
b. Endogenous vasopressin levels are typically low in patients with septic shock.
c. It increases smooth muscle intracellular calcium.
d. Vasopressin infusion is effective in reducing noradrenaline requirements in patients with septic shock.
e. Vasopressin should be infused at a rate of between 1-3 units/min.

5 Regarding delirium in the intensive care patient:

a. Prophylactic haloperidol has been shown to reduce the incidence of delirium in critically ill patients.
b. The Confusion Assessment Method for the ICU (CAM-ICU) test includes assessment of recall, orientation and inattention.
c. Hyperactive delirium is the commonest subtype.
d. Audiovisual reorientation has been shown to benefit patients suffering from delirium.
e. Sedation with a single agent, dexmedetomidine, as compared to benzodiazepines significantly reduces the incidence of post-sedation delirium.

6 Regarding the anatomy of the larynx and trachea:

a. The cricoid cartilage is situated at the level of C4.
b. The cricotracheal membrane is the preferred site for cricothyrotomy.
c. An aortic aneurysm can cause paralysis of the left vocal cord.
d. In an adult the trachea is approximately 10cm long.
e. The anterior jugular vein is at increased risk of damage if a tracheostomy is not performed in the midline.

7 The following are complications of the treatment of diabetic ketoacidosis:

a. Hypomagnesaemia.
b. Cerebral oedema.
c. Hyperphosphatemia.
d. Hyperchloraemic acidosis.
e. Coagulopathy.

8 The following are recognised causes of a normal anion gap metabolic acidosis:

a. Ureteroenterostomy.
b. Administration of excess normal saline solution.
c. Addison's disease.
d. Use of a carbonic anhydrase inhibitor.
e. Diabetic ketoacidosis.

9 Regarding the anatomy of the cardiovascular system:

a. The common carotid artery divides at the level of C4 into the internal and external carotid arteries.
b. Disruption of the superior mesenteric artery causes ischaemia of the ileum.
c. Saphenous vein cut-down is performed where the great saphenous vein passes anterior to the lateral malleolus.
d. The right coronary artery descends between the pulmonary trunk and the right atrium to run in the anterior atrioventricular groove.
e. The anterior spinal artery is formed by the union of the vertebral arteries at the foramen magnum.

10 The following are causes of prolongation of the corrected QT interval (QTc):

a. Atenolol.
b. Hypercalcaemia.
c. Subarachnoid haemorrhage.
d. Hyperthermia.
e. Hypokalaemia.

11 Regarding fluid therapy on the intensive care unit:

a. Human albumin solution is the preferred resuscitation fluid in traumatic brain injury.
b. The use of hydroxyethyl starch has not been shown to increase mortality in critically ill patients.
c. The use of hydroxyethyl starch as a resuscitation fluid has been shown to decrease the incidence of acute kidney injury in patients with sepsis.
d. The FEAST (Fluid Expansion As Supportive Therapy) trial supports the use of a 20ml/kg initial crystalloid bolus strategy in acutely ill children.
e. The SAFE (Saline versus Albumin Fluid Evaluation) study suggests that the use of albumin as a primary resuscitation fluid is generally associated with worse outcomes in critically ill patients.

12 When performing a lumbar puncture:

a. In an adult a lumbar puncture can safely be performed at the level of L2/3.
b. Cerebrospinal fluid is located in the epidural space.
c. When performing a lumbar puncture in the sitting position, a normal opening pressure is 20-40cm of cerebrospinal fluid.
d. Cerebrospinal fluid is formed by the arachnoid villi in the lateral, third and fourth ventricles.
e. Cerebrospinal fluid has an osmolality of approximately 280mOsm/kg.

13 Which of the following are true regarding arterial pressure waveform analysis?

a. The dicrotic notch represents aortic valve closure.
b. Vasoconstriction is suggested by a steep slope of systolic decay.
c. The rate of rise in pressure per unit time (dP/dt) is an index of contractility.

d. A large delta (Δ) down in a ventilated patient suggests hypovolaemia.
e. The stoke volume is derived from the area under the arterial waveform.

14 When using a pulmonary artery catheter, the following are directly measured variables:

a. Left atrial pressure.
b. Cardiac index.
c. Oxygen delivery.
d. Mixed venous SaO_2.
e. Right ventricular systolic pressure.

15 Regarding the mechanism of action of drugs via receptors and second messenger systems:

a. Suxamethonium works on a ligand gated ion channel.
b. Thyroxine works via the tyrosine kinase system.
c. Gi receptors cause an increase in activity of adenylate cyclase.
d. Nitric oxide increases the levels of intracellular cyclic guanosine monophosphate (cGMP).
e. α1-adrenoceptors are Gq proteins.

16 The following may be used to reduce the incidence of clotting in the haemofilter circuit:

a. Reduce the pre-dilution to a post-dilution ratio.
b. Fondaparinux.
c. Albumin.
d. Citrate.
e. Epoprostenol.

17 Concerning the use of the oesophageal Doppler probe for cardiac monitoring in the ICU:

a. The monitor assumes that 70% of total stroke volume enters the descending aorta.
b. Peak velocity can be used as an age-dependent marker of afterload.
c. FTc is corrected to a heart rate of 60bpm.
d. Probe placement is contraindicated in cribriform plate fracture.
e. A high FTc suggests vasoplegia.

18 The dosing schedule of the following antimicrobial agents should be modified in patients with chronic kidney disease (CKD) stage 3:

a. Tazocin.
b. Metronidazole.
c. Meropenem.
d. Amphotericin.
e. Clarithromycin.

19 Regarding posterior circulation ischaemic stroke, which of the following are true?

a. Posterior circulation stroke accounts for 20-25% of ischaemic strokes.
b. Posterior circulation transient ischaemic attacks are easier to diagnose than those of the anterior circulation.
c. Carotid Doppler assessment may be diagnostic.
d. The risk of recurrent stroke after posterior circulation stroke is lower than for anterior circulation stroke.
e. Neurosurgical decompression may be a useful treatment option.

20 With regard to the intra-aortic balloon pump:

a. Balloon inflation is timed to coincide with the dicrotic notch on the aortic waveform trace.
b. Increased afterload leads to increased coronary perfusion pressure.
c. The balloon is inflated with air.
d. The balloon is positioned proximal to the left subclavian artery.
e. Randomised controlled trial data support its use in cardiogenic shock complicating myocardial infarction to decrease 30-day mortality.

21 Regarding arterial blood gas analysis:

a. The pH of a gas sample is directly measured.
b. All arterial blood gas samples are measured at 37°C +/- 0.1°C.
c. The blood gas analyser will underestimate the true *in vivo* $PaCO_2$ of a hypothermic patient.
d. Bubbles of air in the gas syringe will affect the measured PaO_2.
e. Leukopaenia can cause pseudohypoxaemia.

22 A 37-year-old man is assaulted and sustains a severe traumatic brain injury. He undergoes a craniotomy for an extradural haematoma. The neurosurgical team insert an intracranial pressure bolt for intracranial pressure monitoring (ICP). Regarding ICP monitoring;

a. Lundberg A waves are normal.
b. P1 is the percussion wave corresponding to transmission of the venous pressure from the choroid plexus.
c. P2 represents the dicrotic notch correlating with the closure of the aortic valve.
d. When the amplitude of P2 exceeds P1 this is suggestive of reduced brain compliance.
e. Normally ICP increases slightly with each arterial pulse because of transient increases in cerebral blood volume.

23 During a respiratory wean, the following numerical indices suggest a spontaneous breathing trial is likely to be followed by successful extubation:

a. Rapid Shallow Breathing Index (RSBI) <105.
b. Respiratory rate <35/min.
c. Vital capacity >5ml/kg.
d. PO_2 >10kPa.
e. $ETCO_2$ <5kPa.

24 Regarding balloon tamponade devices for the management of variceal bleeding:

a. Sengstaken-Blakemore tubes have two balloon inflation ports and two ports for aspiration.
b. A patient must be intubated with an endotracheal tube *in situ* before a Sengstaken-Blakemore tube is inserted.
c. The oesophageal balloon should be inflated before the gastric balloon.
d. Weighted traction using a bag of saline should be applied to the Sengstaken-Blakemore tube post-insertion.
e. Rebleeding occurs in approximately 50% of patients when the tube is removed if no other intervention has taken place.

25 A 55-year-old man undergoes a 6-hour coronary artery bypass graft procedure on cardiopulmonary bypass. He has a background of Type 1 diabetes mellitus. He took occasional paracetamol pre-operatively. The following are risk factors for the development of acute kidney injury in the postoperative period for this man:

a. His age.
b. His gender.

c. His medication history of paracetamol ingestion.
d. Diabetes mellitus.
e. The length of his operation.

26 The application of continuous positive airway pressure (CPAP) or positive end-expiratory pressure (PEEP) typically leads to:

a. Increased functional residual capacity.
b. A reduction in preload in patients with acute cardiogenic pulmonary oedema.
c. Redistribution of extravascular lung water.
d. Increased cardiac output.
e. Decreased intracranial pressure.

27 Regarding the diagnosis and management of acute spinal cord injury:

a. The neurological 'level' of a spinal cord injury is the lowest level of the spinal cord with normal sensation and motor function on both sides of the body.
b. Patients suffering a high spinal cord injury should be nursed in a 45° position during the acute phase.
c. Due to gastroparesis, enteral feeding should be delayed for 48-72 hours post-injury.
d. 90% of patients with spinal cord injury will develop a deep vein thrombosis.
e. It is safe to use depolarising muscle relaxants 6 weeks following spinal cord injury.

28 A 34-year-old man with a diagnosis of Wolff-Parkinson-White (WPW) syndrome is admitted with palpitations. His ECG shows atrial fibrillation with a narrow QRS complex and a ventricular rate of 180 beats per minute;

his blood pressure is 134/78mmHg. Which of the following options would be appropriate treatment?

a.   Verapamil.
b.   Esmolol.
c.   Digoxin.
d.   Flecainide.
e.   Adenosine.

29 In the patient with major burns:

a.   Selective decontamination of the digestive tract has been demonstrated to reduce the incidence of burn wound infection.
b.   The first half of the fluid requirement as calculated by the Parkland formula should be administered over 12 hours.
c.   Pre-hospital fluid should be subtracted from the fluid requirement as calculated by the Parkland formula.
d.   Erythematous areas should be included in the total body surface area (TBSA) calculation.
e.   The modified Baux score can be used to predict mortality.

30 Regarding the acute management of ischaemic stroke:

a.   The ROSIER score predicts the risk of a patient who has suffered a transient ischaemic attack developing a stroke.
b.   The National Institutes of Health Stroke Scale is used to quantify impairment caused by a stroke.
c.   Prophylactic low-molecular-weight heparin should be started in immobile patients to decrease the risk of deep vein thrombosis.
d.   A 72-year-old patient with malignant middle cerebral artery infarction should be considered for decompressive hemicraniectomy to improve the chances of survival.
e.   Aspirin and statin therapy should be given as soon as possible following diagnosis.

31 Which of the following are expected following a significant overdose of amitriptyline?

a. Metabolic acidosis.
b. Seizures.
c. Hyperthermia.
d. Hypocapnia.
e. Urinary retention.

32 The following poisons are correctly matched with potential antidotes:

a. Methanol = fomepizole.
b. Cyanide = sodium thiosulphate.
c. β-blockade = salbutamol.
d. Organophosphates = pralidoxime.
e. Paraquat = oxygen.

33 Regarding methods for assessing and measuring quality of life in the intensive care population:

a. A quality-adjusted life-year (QALY) is the arithmetic product of life expectancy and a measure of the quality of the remaining life-years.
b. The smallest possible value of a QALY is 0, which is equivalent to death.
c. EQ-5D is an objective measure of quality of life.
d. The Hospital Anxiety and Depression Scale is a subjective measure of quality of life.
e. The Medical Outcome Short Form Health Survey (SF-36) measures 36 items to determine quality of life.

34 An 18-year-old female is admitted to the ICU with a fever of 39°C and a maculopapular rash. Her blood pressure is refractory to fluid resuscitation and her systolic blood pressure remains 80mmHg after 4L of fluid. The admitting physician suspects toxic shock syndrome (TSS). Regarding this condition:

a. It is usually caused by a retained vaginal tampon.
b. An elevated serum creatinine phosphokinase (CPK) is a diagnostic feature.
c. Mucous membrane involvement is typical.
d. The majority of cases occur in females.
e. TSS may be the presenting feature of leptospirosis.

35 The following initial therapeutic measures are supported by level I evidence in the presence of new-onset acute upper GI bleeding:

a. A transfusion trigger of 70g/L haemoglobin.
b. Empirical administration of broad-spectrum antibiotics in patients with cirrhotic liver disease.
c. Terlipressin in patients with known or suspected varices.
d. Minnesota tube placement.
e. Proton pump inhibition.

36 The following principles are true regarding the end of life care of intensive care patients in the UK:

a. Any management plan specifying limits of invasive interventions must be reviewed daily.
b. Unanimity amongst the medical and nursing team is necessary before withdrawal of life-sustaining treatment can take place.
c. The healthcare professional responsible for making the decision about the extent of treatment in a patient lacking capacity should consult with those close to the patient to help reach a decision.
d. Should an Independent Mental Capacity Advocate be appointed, they assume the responsibility of making the final decision about withdrawal.
e. A legally binding advance care plan which includes requests for specific treatments must be honoured by the treating medical team.

37 A 58-year-old woman is admitted with community-acquired pneumonia. She has a past medical history of diabetes and asthma and is previously independent. She is hypotensive with a blood pressure of 90/40mmHg and tachycardic with a heart rate of 135 beats per minute in the resuscitation room of the emergency department. Which of the following are true statements regarding initial management?

a. Initial fluid bolus should be colloid.
b. Broad-spectrum antibiotics should be given within the first 6 hours of recognition of septic shock.
c. Fluid therapy should be titrated to base excess.
d. Vasopressin is the preferred first-line vasopressor.
e. Initial fluid challenge should be 30ml/kg.

38 The following are components of the CAM-ICU delirium screening tool:

a. Variation in sedation score in the last 24 hours.
b. Ingestion of deliriogenic medication in the last 24 hours.
c. Evidence of inattention on testing.
d. Abbreviated mental test score <6.
e. Non-compliance with therapy in the last 24 hours.

39 Regarding the logistics of organ donation:

a. Functional warm ischaemic time begins with the onset of asystole.
b. Cold ischaemic time is the time from initiation of cold preservation until the restoration of warm circulation after transplant.
c. Age >80 years is a contraindication to organ donation.
d. A donation after cardiac death (DCD) patient is not suitable for heart donation.
e. Noradrenaline is the first-line agent for the management of fluid-resistant hypotension in the brainstem-dead donor.

40 A 56-year-old male is admitted with severe sepsis. His blood cultures have grown Gram-positive bacteria. Which of the following are examples of Gram-positive bacteria?

a. *Bacillus.*
b. *Streptococci.*
c. *Clostridium.*
d. *Haemophilus.*
e. *Listeria.*

41 The following are recognised causes of isotonic hyponatraemia:

a. Hyperglycaemia.
b. The syndrome of inappropriate antidiuretic hormone secretion (SIADH).
c. Glycine absorption during urological surgery.
d. Addison's disease.
e. Beer potomania.

42 When considering the repatriation of a critically ill patient by air transfer, the following should be borne in mind:

a. The change in volume of a mass of gas is directly proportional to the change in atmospheric pressure during an air transfer.
b. When flying at altitude, endotracheal cuffs must be filled with saline.
c. Defibrillation at normal energy levels can be undertaken without risk to the aircraft or crew.
d. Patients with decompression sickness are not suitable for air transfer.
e. Acceleration forces experienced in routine helicopter operations are similar to those experienced in road transfers.

43 A 45-year-old man is extricated out of the local canal after drowning. He has severe hypothermia. Which of these features would be expected on his ECG?

a. A negative deflection at the junction of the QRS and ST segments in the chest leads.
b. Atrial fibrillation.
c. Short PR interval.
d. Bradyarrhythmia.
e. Ventricular ectopics.

44 The following are recommended initial treatment options in the management of severe symptomatic hypotonic hyponatraemia of indeterminate onset:

a. Administration of 3% hypertonic saline.
b. Desmopressin.
c. Conivaptan.
d. Demeclocycline.
e. Fludrocortisone.

45 Regarding infection control and methods of cleaning equipment:

a. According to the World Health Organization "Your 5 Moments for Hand Hygiene", hands should be cleaned after touching any objects in the patient's immediate surroundings.
b. Matching Michigan was a patient safety initiative to decrease the incidence of ventilator-associated pneumonia.
c. Using 2% chlorhexidine in 70% isopropyl alcohol for skin preparation sterilises the skin prior to central venous catheter insertion.
d. Pulse oximeter probes must be decontaminated between patients.

e. Any item which comes into contact with mucous membranes must be disinfected before subsequent use.

46 Which of the following are features of acute aortic dissection on a plain chest X-ray?

a. Pleural capping.
b. Right-sided pleural effusion.
c. Calcium sign.
d. Depression of right main bronchus.
e. Tracheal shift.

47 Regarding the patient with necrotising fasciitis:

a. Type 2 is of fungal aetiology.
b. Most infections are single-organism clostridial species.
c. Clindamycin is usually recommended as empirical Gram-negative coverage.
d. Scoring systems based on laboratory values can usefully distinguish between necrotising fasciitis and other soft tissue infections.
e. Standard care includes hyperbaric oxygen therapy.

48 The following infectious diseases are notifiable to local authority proper officers:

a. Haemolytic uraemic syndrome.
b. Tetanus.
c. Acute viral meningitis.
d. Tuberculosis.
e. Acute hepatitis C infection.

49 A 45-year-old male sustains a crush injury to his leg in a road traffic accident and has a comminuted tibial fracture. He develops a swollen tense leg. The possibility of acute compartment syndrome in his leg is considered. Regarding this condition:

a. Pain is exacerbated by passive stretching.
b. Palpable distal pulses make the diagnosis unlikely.
c. In the leg, the most commonly affected compartment is the posterior compartment.
d. Capillary blood flow in the compartment is typically compromised once the tissue pressure exceeds diastolic blood pressure.
e. Patients with a coagulopathy are at risk of developing this condition.

50 In a patient with suspected acute kidney injury (AKI) on the intensive care unit:

a. Serum and urinary neutrophil gelatinase-associated lipoprotein (NGAL) are likely to rise prior to serum creatinine.
b. N-acetyl cysteine may limit progression to chronic renal failure if administered early.
c. A urine output <0.5ml/kg/hr for more than 6 hours confirms the first stage of AKI as per the RIFLE criteria.
d. Progression to chronic kidney disease (CKD) is defined as a glomerular filtration rate (GFR) persistently <60ml/min for a period of at least 3 months.
e. The use of hydroxyethyl starch as a resuscitation fluid has shown evidence of benefit in reducing the incidence of acute kidney injury in critically ill patients.

51 Regarding electricity, electrical safety and the pathophysiological effects of electricity:

a. Resistance is greatest when the potential difference is high and the current is low.

b.   The resistance of skin is decreased ten-fold when it becomes wet.
c.   The risk of ventricular fibrillation is greatest if the electric current passes through the myocardium during the depolarisation of the myocardial cells.
d.   A 5mA current passing from hand to hand is sufficient to cause ventricular fibrillation.
e.   A piece of equipment with a leakage current of <500µA can safely be attached to a pulmonary artery catheter.

52 Regarding the diagnosis of diabetic ketoacidosis (DKA), the following diagnostic criteria apply:

a.   Plasma bicarbonate >15mmol/L.
b.   Venous pH <7.3.
c.   Serum osmolarity ≥320mOsm/kg.
d.   Blood glucose >20mmol/L.
e.   Ketonuria.

53 With regard to acute severe pancreatitis:

a.   The revised Atlanta classification defines pancreatitis as at least two of the following: a serum lipase/amylase >5 times the upper limit of normal; radiological evidence of pancreatic inflammation; consistent abdominal symptoms.
b.   An APACHE II score >8 or a Glasgow score >3 within the first 24 hours are strongly predictive of complications and suggestive of the need for critical care support.
c.   The Marshall severity scoring system uses a computed tomography severity index to provide radiological grading of pancreatitis severity and extension.
d.   The Balthazar grading system incorporates assessment of renal cardiovascular and respiratory indices.
e.   Serum lipase is a preferred initial diagnostic test, due to its superior sensitivity and specificity.

54 Regarding the mode of action of oral and parenteral anticoagulants:

a. Dabigatran is a direct thrombin inhibitor.
b. Bivalirudin is a direct Factor Xa inhibitor.
c. Danaparoid is an indirect Factor Xa inhibitor.
d. Fondaparinux is an indirect thrombin inhibitor.
e. Rivaroxiban is a direct thrombin inhibitor.

55 A 54-year-old patient is sedated and ventilated for respiratory failure due to pneumonia. She is successfully extubated but develops severe dyspnoea and diaphoresis a few hours later. Following urgent echocardiography a diagnosis of Takotsubo cardiomyopathy (TCM) is considered. Regarding TCM:

a. It affects males more commonly than females.
b. It may be triggered by an emotionally or stressful event.
c. The ECG is usually normal.
d. Septal ballooning on transthoracic echocardiography is typical.
e. Coronary angiography is a useful investigation.

56 With regard to POSSUM scoring:

a. The POSSUM scoring system accurately predicts risk of death for individual patients undergoing major surgery.
b. The general model includes only physiological and intra-operative parameters.
c. Versions of the POSSUM score are available for vascular, general and oesophagogastric patients.
d. ECG findings are included as a physiological parameter.
e. Urine output is included as a postoperative parameter.

57 Regarding the use of humidification and nebulisers on the intensive care unit:

a. When air is inhaled it is fully humidified and warmed by the patient's nasopharynx by the time it enters the trachea.
b. Heat and moisture exchangers typically deliver air with a relative humidity of 90%.
c. A hot water humidifier can achieve a relative humidity of 100% at 37°C.
d. The use of an ultrasonic nebuliser in a ventilated patient may impair ventilator triggering.
e. In a ventilated patient approximately 50% of the nebuliser charge is lost due to aerosol deposition in the ventilator circuit, endotracheal tube and large conducting airways.

58 Regarding rhabdomyolysis:

a. It can be caused by carbon monoxide poisoning.
b. Myoglobin precipitates in renal tubules causing obstruction.
c. Mannitol reduces the risk of renal failure.
d. Alkanisation of urine increases cast formation.
e. Hypocalcaemia should be aggressively corrected.

59 A 75-year-old lady is admitted to the ITU following debridement of necrotising fasciitis. On day 7 her bloods and gas show the following picture: Na^+ 146mmol/L, Cl^- 113mmol/L, K^+ 4.6mmol/L, urea 19mmol/L, albumin 6g/L, pH 7.45, pCO_2 5.1, bicarbonate 27mmol/L, BE +3.3mEq/L:

a. There is an element of hyperchloraemic acidosis.
b. There is an element of hypoalbuminaemic acidosis.
c. Hypernatraemia will cause a metabolic alkalosis.

d. The strong ion difference (SID) is 33meq/L.
e. There is no significant physiological disturbance.

60 Regarding the diagnosis and management of hypertension:

a. Diagnosis requires elevated blood pressure measurement on three separate occasions.
b. Stage 2 hypertension is defined as a systolic BP >159mmHg and/or a diastolic BP >99mmHg.
c. Resistant hypertension is defined as a blood pressure greater than 140/90mmHg despite optimal doses of three antihypertensive agents.
d. Hypertensive urgency describes severe hypertension with evidence of end-organ damage.
e. Patients with severe, asymptomatic hypertension should have their BP quickly lowered to less than 140/90mmHg.

Single best answer questions — select ONE answer from the five choices

61 A 67-year-old man suffers a cardiopulmonary arrest on a surgical ward. He is in ventricular fibrillation. The arrest team are struggling to site intravenous access. The anaesthetist has intubated him and he has received two DC shocks. Cardiopulmonary resuscitation is in progress. According to the 2010 Advanced Life Support (ALS) Resuscitation Guidance the preferred strategy for drug administration would be:

a. Insertion of an intraosseous needle.
b. Intramuscular administration of drugs.
c. Administration of drugs via the endotracheal tube.
d. Surgical cutdown and cannulation of the long saphenous vein.
e. Insertion of a central venous catheter by a competent operator under ultrasound guidance.

62 Which of the following patients would be most likely to benefit from venovenous extracorporeal membrane oxygenation (VV ECMO)?

a. A 65-year-old post-ST-elevation myocardial infarction (STEMI) with cardiogenic shock and refractory hypoxaemia.
b. A 35-year-old with worsening idiopathic pulmonary fibrosis and acute hospital-acquired pneumonia.
c. A 45-year-old male out-of-hospital cardiac arrest (suspected cardiac aetiology) following 45 minutes of advanced life support and intermittent return of spontaneous circulation.
d. A 60-year-old lung transplant patient with early graft failure and refractory hypoxaemia.
e. A 30-year-old renal transplant patient with end-stage vascular access who has now developed *Cytomegalovirus* (CMV) pneumonitis and refractory hypercarbia on ventilation.

63 An 89-year-old man is found on the floor of his house. There is evidence of severe diarrhoea and vomiting. He is confused and complaining of lethargy and tingling of his hands and feet. While being transferred to hospital he suffers a brief, self-terminating seizure. On arrival, examination shows muscle weakness with positive Chovstek's and Trousseau's signs. ECG shows ST depression, T-wave flattening and U-waves, and a QTc of 500ms. Which primary electrolyte disturbance best explains all these findings?

a. Hypokalaemia.
b. Hypocalcaemia.
c. Hyponatraemia.
d. Hypercalcaemia.
e. Hypomagnesaemia.

64 A 75-year-old man is admitted to the emergency department with confusion and photophobia. His family report that he has been generally unwell and lethargic for a week and has had diarrhoea. He is pyrexial at 38.9°C. His white cell count is 18.0 x 10³/ml. Lumbar puncture is performed. Cerebrospinal fluid (CSF) analysis reveals a pleocytosis, and CSF protein levels are moderately elevated at 0.80g/L. CSF glucose is 1.3mmol/L. The Gram stain is negative. The most likely diagnosis is:

a.   *Neisseria* meningitis.
b.   Subdural haematoma.
c.   *Listeria* meningitis.
d.   Viral meningitis.
e.   Cryptococcal meningitis.

65 You are asked to review a 45-year-old man on the ICU with refractory hypoxia. He was admitted several days ago with acute pancreatitis and has subsequently developed severe acute respiratory distress syndrome. His PEEP and FiO_2 have been escalated over the course of the day. He is now saturating at 85% on FiO_2 0.65 with PEEP at 15cm H_2O and plateau pressures of 29cm H_2O. There is little to remove on tracheal suction. He is sedated and paralysed and the I:E ratio is currently 1:1. Which of the following options would be the most effective next step?

a.   Commencing inhaled nitric oxide.
b.   Adjusting the PEEP to 20cm H_2O in line with the ARDSnet high PEEP ladder.
c.   Placing the patient in the prone position.
d.   Inverting the I:E ratio.
e.   Commencing high-frequency oscillatory ventilation.

66 A 24-year-old 75kg man is brought in by ambulance to the emergency room having been found in a local park. On examination he is found to have a large left-sided groin abscess. Observations include a temperature of 35°C, heart rate (HR) 139bpm and a mean arterial pressure (MAP) of 47mmHg. His serum lactate is 4.3mmol/L. Bloods show a haemoglobin concentration of 94g/L and a white cell count of 21 x 10^9/L. He is given an initial bolus of 2L of Hartmann's solution, his MAP improves to 52mmHg and his HR decreases to 124bpm. The most appropriate next step from the list below is:

a. Noradrenaline infusion.
b. Further crystalloid administration.
c. Transfusion of packed red cells.
d. Administration of a starch for fluid resuscitation.
e. Transfer to theatre for immediate wound debridement.

67 A 79-year-old man is on the coronary care unit at a peripheral hospital after an inferior ST elevation myocardial infarction (STEMI) which was too late a presentation to consider transfer for primary coronary intervention. He deteriorates in the early hours one morning with chest pain and a drop in blood pressure. BP is 90/52mmHg. He has had slow intravenous fluid running. His jugular venous pressure is elevated and chest is clear. Which of the following is the most appropriate course of action?

a. Re-referral to the local cardiac centre.
b. Intravenous nitrates.
c. Stop intravenous fluids.
d. Intravenous furosemide.
e. Thrombolysis.

68 Which of the following qualities is most essential when designing a scoring system to assess risk of mortality in critically ill patients?

a. Validity.
b. Generalisabilty.
c. Complexity of statistical modelling.
d. Discrimination.
e. Simplicity of variables.

69 A 54-year-old woman is admitted to hospital following ingestion of an unknown substance 14 hours previously. She is acting strangely and complaining of visual disturbances, nausea and abdominal pain. On examination her observations are as follows: GCS 14, HR 118bpm, BP 89/54mmHg, respiratory rate 30/min. Urine toxicology is negative for amphetamines, barbiturates, benzodiazepines and opiates. Blood results: serum Na^+ 139mmol/L, serum K^+ 4.3mmol/L, serum urea 6.5mmol/L, serum creatinine 105μmol/L, Cl^- 106mmol/L, blood glucose 5.8mmol/L, serum osmolarity 312mOsm/L. Paracetamol and salicylate levels are awaited. Arterial blood gas (on air): pH 7.15, pO_2 13.1kPa, pCO_2 2.1kPa, HCO_3^- 7mmol/L. No abnormalities are seen on chest X-ray. ECG shows sinus tachycardia, QRS duration 100ms. What is the most likely intoxicant?

a. Ethylene glycol.
b. Salicylates.
c. Tricyclic antidepressants.
d. Cyanide.
e. Paraquat.

70 A 23-year-old lady who is 32 weeks' pregnant presents to the hospital with severe vomiting. Her blood pressure is 168/110mmHg. She has no headache and no visual disturbances. Liver function tests reveal bilirubin of 165µmol/L, aspartate aminotransferase of 700IU/L, fibrinogen 0.5g/L and a prothrombin time of 29 seconds. Her plasma glucose is 2.3mmol/L. Which of the following is the most likely diagnosis?

a. Acute fatty liver of pregnancy.
b. Liver haematoma.
c. Veno-occlusive disease.
d. Cholestasis of pregnancy.
e. Viral hepatitis.

71 A 25-year-old male is admitted to the intensive care unit with meningococcal sepsis. On arrival he has a lactate of 5mmol/L, a pulse of 160bpm and a blood pressure of 76/25mmHg. Capillary refill time is 5 seconds. He has been intubated in the emergency department and has central access. He has been resuscitated with 4L of crystalloid fluid. His estimated weight is 72kg. He has warm peripheries and bounding pulses. From the following options, what would be the next recommended measure?

a. Hydrocortisone infusion.
b. Further fluid bolus with 20ml/kg 4.5% human albumin solution.
c. Intravenous vasopressin infusion.
d. Intravenous noradrenaline infusion.
e. Further crystalloid boluses until lactate <2mmol/L.

Paper 2 Questions

72 A 40-year-old 41-week pregnant female is 6cm dilated following spontaneous onset of labour. She has had 2 previous live births by normal vaginal delivery. She starts complaining of a headache and chest pain, and rapidly becomes hypotensive, tachypnoeic and tachycardic. Cardiotocography (CTG) shows foetal distress. Her oxygen saturations drop to 83% on air and over the next 30 minutes she is noted to be oozing from one of her drip sites. Her GCS drops to 3 and she has a brief tonic-clonic seizure. Bloods show haemoglobin 95g/L, platelets 84 x 10^9/L, APTT 54 seconds, prothombin time 23 seconds, fibrinogen 1.1g/L. Arterial blood gas shows pH 7.3, pO_2 6.4kPa, pCO_2 4.0kPa, HCO_3^- 14mmol/L. No abnormality is seen on chest X-ray. ECG shows a right ventricular strain pattern. The most appropriate diagnosis is:

a.   Sepsis.
b.   Pulmonary embolism.
c.   Amniotic fluid embolism.
d.   Placental abruption.
e.   Eclampsia.

73 A 56-year-old woman is admitted with sudden onset of shortness of breath and haemoptysis. Her blood pressure is 120/67mmHg. She has a history of a recent long haul travel. A diagnosis of pulmonary embolism (PE) is considered and subsequently confirmed by CT pulmonary angiogram. An ECG on this patient is most likely to show:

a.   S1Q3T3.
b.   Right axis deviation.
c.   Right bundle branch block (RBBB).

d.   Sinus tachycardia.
e.   Right ventricular hypertrophy.

74 A 70-year-old man is admitted to the unit following a laparotomy for faecal peritonitis. The anaesthetist reports a stormy peri-operative episode, with prolonged periods of hypotension following induction and eventual stabilisation on high-dose adrenaline infusion. During the operation it was noted that his T-waves had become inverted on the cardiac monitor and ECG confirmed this in leads V2-V6. A high sensitivity troponin was sent on closure and has come back at 174ng/mL. Baseline troponin measurements were normal. Focused echo on the unit notes global left ventricular systolic dysfunction. Which of the following is the likely diagnosis for his ECG and biochemical findings?

a.   A Type 1 myocardial infarction.
b.   A Type 2 myocardial infarction.
c.   A Type 3 myocardial infarction.
d.   A Type 4 myocardial infarction.
e.   A Type 5 myocardial infarction.

75 A 44-year-old 60kg woman is admitted to the intensive care unit intubated and ventilated after being admitted with community-acquired pneumonia. She remains intubated and ventilated 48 hours later. She is on 70% oxygen, receiving a 0.02μg/kg/min noradrenaline infusion, full enteral feed and she is sedated with propofol and fentanyl. Regarding prophylaxis for stress ulcers the most appropriate management plan is:

a. Omeprazole.
b. Ranitidine.
c. Sucralfate.
d. Enteral magnesium alginate.
e. No prophylaxis required.

76 A 44-year-old man is admitted with chest pain and agitation. He admits to cocaine use the same day. He has ST segment elevation on his ECG in leads V1-V4. He has a past medical history of smoking, hypertension and hyperlipidaemia. He has a blood pressure of 200/120mmHg. Which of the following is the best immediate management?

a. Intravenous phenoxybenzamine.
b. Urgent CT angiogram.
c. Administer intravenous β-blockers.
d. Urgent thrombolysis.
e. Sedate the patient.

77 An 85-year-old man is admitted to the ICU unit following elective bowel resection. He has known severe aortic stenosis with a peak transvalvular gradient of 80mmHg. The best management of his cardiovascular system would be:

a. Dobutamine to target a high DO_2.
b. ACE-inhibitor therapy to reduce left ventricular remodelling.
c. Hydralazine infusion to decrease afterload.
d. Noradrenaline infusion to increase systemic vascular resistance.
e. Intravenous nitrates to maximise coronary perfusion.

78 An 82-year-old male is admitted through the emergency department with an acute abdomen. He has a past medical history of hypertension, ischaemic heart disease and Type 2 diabetes mellitus. His ECG shows atrial fibrillation, left axis deviation and left ventricular hypertrophy. An echocardiogram performed 2 years previously showed left ventricular hypertrophy with an ejection fraction of 40% and severe tricuspid regurgitation. He undergoes emergency laparotomy where a right hemi-colectomy is performed. Postoperatively, he is intubated and ventilated on the intensive care unit. He becomes increasingly haemodynamically unstable and the decision is made to instigate cardiac output monitoring. What would be the best method of advanced haemodynamic monitoring to employ in this patient?

a. Pulmonary artery catheter.
b. Stroke volume variation.
c. Bioreactance.
d. Oesophageal Doppler.
e. Central venous pressure measurement.

79 An 18-year-old woman is admitted with a 2-week history of a sore throat and headache. She is pyrexial at 38°C. She has deranged liver function tests and splenomegaly on examination. Which of the following tests is most likely to prove diagnostic?

a. Lumbar puncture and urgent Gram stain.
b. CT head.
c. Blood cultures.
d. Monospot test.
e. Abdominal ultrasound scan.

80 A young patient on the unit has an unexplained metabolic acidosis and has been on a large dose of propofol for the last 3 days. The diagnosis of propofol infusion syndrome (PRIS) is considered. Which of the following features is most consistent with this?

a. Widespread T-wave inversion.
b. Bradycardia.
c. High transaminase levels.
d. Jaundice.
e. Fast atrial fibrillation.

81 A 71-year-old woman is admitted to hospital with diarrhoea having been discharged from hospital 15 days previously following treatment (metronidazole) for *Clostridium difficile* infection (CDI). Past medical history includes hypertension, ischaemic heart disease, and Type 2 diabetes mellitus. She also had a CDI 3 months previously, which was also treated with metronidazole. She is having 5-7 stools per day, (Bristol Stool Chart Type 6), which are positive for *C. difficile* toxin. Examination and investigations show: heart rate 95, blood pressure 108/76mmHg, temperature 38°C, serum creatinine 94μmol/L, white cell count 12 x 10^9/L. The most appropriate therapy is:

a. Oral metronidazole 400mg tds.
b. Oral vancomycin 125mg tds.
c. Faecal transplant.
d. Oral fidaxomicin 200mg bd.
e. Oral rifampicin 300mg bd.

82 Which of the following interventions has shown the most potential benefit in reducing the rate of contrast-induced nephropathy (CIN) in critically ill patients with acute kidney injury undergoing CT imaging with contrast?

a. Intravenous crystalloid loading.
b. Intravenous N-acetyl cysteine.
c. Use of a D1 receptor agonist.
d. Low-dose dopamine infusion.
e. Use of high osmolal contrast agents.

83 An 84-year-old female has undergone coronary artery bypass grafting and mitral valve repair. Five hours post-surgery she is managed on the cardiac intensive care unit. She is intubated and ventilated using intermittent positive pressure ventilation and managed on intravenous infusions of milrinone and noradrenaline. She becomes progressively more tachycardic. Repeat observations and cardiac output studies show: HR 143 beats per minute, MAP 65mmHg, central venous pressure (CVP) 20mmHg, CI- 1.4L/min/m^2, systemic vascular resistance index (SVRI) 2800 dyne/s/cm^5/m^2, pulmonary artery occlusion pressure 19mmHg, temperature 37.6°C, drain output 40ml over the last hour. The arterial line shows a pulse pressure variation of >20%. Repeat chest X-ray shows no abnormalities. Given these results, what is the most likely diagnosis?

a. Pulmonary embolism.
b. Haemorrhage.
c. Cardiogenic shock.
d. Tamponade.
e. Tension pneumothorax.

84 A 46-year-old woman's house is set alight by her chip pan. She is trapped in her bedroom for up to 2 hours. The ICU physician is asked to assess her in the emergency department resuscitation room. She has singed nasal hairs and a hoarse voice. She has 40% burns to her torso and extremities and is agitated and in pain. Which of the following is the best option in terms of airway management?

a. Rapid sequence induction and tracheal intubation.
b. Awake fibreoptic intubation.
c. Observe on a high dependency unit.
d. Perform an elective tracheostomy.
e. Trial of continuous positive airway pressure ventilation.

85 A 91-year-old man falls in the garden and sustains fractures to ribs 4-6 on the right side and a small pneumothorax which is managed conservatively. He has no other associated injuries and there is no evidence of myocardial or pulmonary contusions. His past medical history includes ischaemic heart disease, previous myocardial infarction and chronic obstructive pulmonary disease (COPD). His medication includes aspirin and clopidogrel. He is managed on the surgical ward for 24 hours, and then a request is made for assistance with analgesia. In addition to the regular paracetamol and NSAID analgesia he is already receiving which of the following options would be the best choice for pain management in this patient?

a. Paravertebral block.
b. Intercostal nerve blocks.
c. Thoracic epidural.
d. Entonox®.
e. Change from oral to intravenous paracetamol.

86 A long-stay patient develops hypophosphataemia, hypomagnesaemia and hypokalaemia following the introduction of enteral nutrition. What is the most appropriate next management step?

a. Electrolyte replacement and continue enteral feeding.
b. Electrolyte replacement and stop enteral feeding.
c. Electrolyte replacement and reduce enteral feeding.
d. Electrolyte replacement and convert enteral feed to parenteral nutrition.
e. Potassium replacement, continue enteral feeding and allow shift of other electrolytes from total body stores to render equilibrium.

87 A 76-year-old nursing home resident is admitted to hospital in a confused state. On examination the patient is found to be hyperreflexic with a GCS of 9. She is tachycardic and hypotensive with dry mucous membranes but maintains a good urine output. Bloods show serum Na^+ 171mmol/L, K^+ 2.8mmol/L, serum glucose 12mmol/L and serum osmolality 310mOsm/kg. Urinalysis shows osmolality 272mOsm/kg. Once the patient is stabilised and her serum sodium returned to normal a water deprivation test is performed. Prior to the test her urine osmolality is 275mOsm/kg, after water deprivation urine osmolality is 274mOsm/kg and after the administration of desmopressin, urine osmolality is 270mOsm/kg. The most likely diagnosis is.

a. Primary hyperaldosteronism.
b. Cushing's syndrome.
c. Nephrogenic diabetes insipidus.
d. Central diabetes insipidus.
e. Hypodipsia.

88 A 27-year-old man is bought into the emergency department by ambulance complaining of shortness of breath. He has a history of asthma and takes salbutamol and beclometasone inhalers regularly. Which of the following examination findings would be the most worrying clinical sign?

a. Heart rate of 125/minute.
b. Speaking in short sentences due to breathlessness.
c. Respiratory rate of 28/minute.
d. Peak expiratory flow rate of 40% predicted.
e. Blood pressure of 80/60mmHg.

89 You are managing a patient with a World Federation of Neurosurgeons (WFNS) grade 3 subarachnoid haemorrhage post-coiling, who is now at day 7. Today they have developed a dense left-sided weakness. The neurosurgical team suspects vasospasm. Which of the following options is most likely to be of benefit?

a. Intravenous high-dose nifedipine.
b. Aggressive fluid loading aiming for hypervolaemia and a supranormal CVP.
c. Induced hypertension aiming to increase MAP by 10-20%.
d. Haemodilution to a haematocrit of 0.23.
e. Prescription of high-dose atorvastatin.

90 You are asked to review a 58-year-old 90kg man on the medical ward. He was admitted 24 hours previously with a 3-week history of fatigue, anorexia, weight loss, pyrexia and abdominal pain. His past medical history includes a history of hypertension, kidney stones and a recent course of antibiotics for a urinary tract infection. Bloods show an acute rise in serum creatinine to 2.5 times his baseline and he has passed 80ml urine over the last 4 hours. His fractional excretion of sodium is 4% and coarse granular casts and renal tubular epithelial cell casts are seen on urine microscopy. There are no red cell or white cell casts or eosinophils. The most likely pathophysiology is:

a. Hypovolaemia.
b. Acute tubular necrosis.
c. Acute glomerulonephritis.
d. Urinary tract obstruction.
e. Acute interstitial nephritis.

Paper 2
Answers

F, F, F, T, T

Intensive care unit-acquired weakness (ICUAW) is a clinically detected weakness in critically ill patients where there is no plausible aetiology other than critical illness. Patients with ICUAW are subsequently classified into those with critical illness polyneuropathy (CIP), critical illness myopathy (CIM), or critical illness neuromyopathy (CINM) based on electrophysiological studies. CIM can be further subclassified histologically into cachectic myopathy, thick filament myopathy, and necrotising myopathy.

Approximately 46% of the patients with severe sepsis, multiple organ failure, or prolonged mechanical ventilation will develop ICUAW. Other risk factors include hyperglycaemia, increasing duration of the inflammatory response and increasing duration of multi-organ failure. Other associations include: age; female gender; high severity of illness on admission; hypoalbuminaemia and the use of renal replacement therapy, vasopressors and corticosteroids.

The primary management is aimed at identifying and minimising risk factors, good glucose control and optimising rehabilitation with a multidisciplinary approach to care.

. Appleton R, Kinsella J. Intensive care unit-acquired weakness. *Contin Educ Anaesth Crit Care Pain* 2012; 12: 62-6.

43

2   F, T, T, T, F

Scoring systems are used in critical care as diagnostic and prognostic tools, as well as to guide therapy and management decisions. We are also heavily reliant on them for data collection and assessment. It is essential to be familiar with the common systems in use and to have an understanding of their caveats and validity.

There are currently four versions of the APACHE score — the latter requires paid subscription for use of the mathematical model and as such is not commonly used throughout the UK. Disease-specific scoring systems address the likelihood of either a positive diagnosis or deterioration in a specific condition. The 4T score assesses the pretest probability of heparin-induced thrombocytopaenia, the Blatchford score looks at severity of upper GI bleeding and the Wells prediction rules look at the likelihood of venous thromboembolic disease.

The SOFA score is different to the APACHE and other measures of acute physiology in that it has been validated for sequential use and assessment to determine the likelihood of response to treatment. The Abbreviated Injury Scale (AIS), Injury Severity Score (ISS) and Revised Trauma Score (RTS) have all been previously utilised to assess the severity of traumatic injury on admission to hospital and to code as major trauma. The RASS is a 9-point scale used as a marker of sedation on the majority of UK intensive care units. The Ramsay Sedation Scale has 5 points.

1. Knaus WA, Wagner DP, Draper EA, *et al*. The APACHE III prognostic system. Risk prediction of hospital mortality for critically ill hospitalized adults. *Chest* 1991; 100(6): 1619-36.
2. Ferreira FL, Bota DP, Bross A, *et al*. Serial evaluation of the SOFA score to predict outcome in critically ill patients. *JAMA* 2001; 286(14): 1754-8.
3. Vincent JL, Moreno R. Scoring systems in the critically ill. *Crit Care* 2010; 14: 207-14.
3. http://www.icudelirium.org/docs/RASS.pdf (accessed 26th July 2014).

3   F, F, F, T, F

There are four phases of trials for new medications. Phase 1 trials aim to test the safety of a new medicine in a small number of people for the first time, who may be healthy volunteers. Phase 2 trials test the new medicine on a larger group of people who are ill. Phase 3 trials test medicines in larger groups of people who are ill, and compare new medicines against an existing treatment of placebo. Phase 4 trials take place once new medicines have been given a marketing licence. The safety, side effects and effectiveness of the medicine continue to be studied while it is being used in practice.

The World Health Organization and the Cochrane Collaboration are amongst those organisations who have adopted the use of GRADE (Grading of Recommendations, Assessment, Development and Evaluation). The GRADE system classifies the quality of evidence into high, moderate, low and very low categories. Evidence based on randomised controlled trials (RCTs) begins as high quality evidence, but confidence in the evidence may be decreased by study limitations, inconsistency of results, indirectness of evidence, imprecision and reporting bias. The GRADE system offers only two grades of recommendations: strong and weak.

A Type I error (α) occurs when the null hypothesis is rejected when it is actually true. A Type II error (β) occurs when we do not reject the null hypothesis when there is, in fact, a difference between the groups. The power of a study is defined as $1-\beta$ and is the probability of rejecting the null hypothesis when it is false. The power of a study is calculated during the planning phase of a study, usually to ensure that the sample size is sufficiently large to give the study sufficient power. Blood pressure is an example of quantitative, continuous data with a normal distribution. Therefore, parametric tests should be utilised to anaylse the data.

1. Clinical trials and medical research - phases of trials. NHS Choices. http://www.nhs.uk/Conditions/Clinical-trials/Pages/Phasesoftrials.aspx (accessed 2nd August 2014).
2. Guyatt GH, Oxman AD, Vist GE, et al. GRADE: an emerging consensus on rating quality of evidence and strength of recommendations. Br Med J 2008; 336: 924-6.
3. Swinscow TDV. Statistics at Square One, 9th ed. London, UK: BMJ Publishing Group, 1997.

4   F, T, T, T, F

Vasopressin is synthesised in the hypothalamus and secreted from the posterior pituitary. Vasopressin infusion has been proven to have a noradrenaline-sparing effect. Endogenous levels of vasopressin may be appropriately high with the first 6 hours in patients with septic shock, but may subsequently fall due to exhaustion of stores, suppression with high-dose noradrenaline or dysfunction of the autonomic nervous system. There is, therefore, a biological rationale for supplementing endogenous vasopressin with an infusion.

The actions of vasopressin are mediated by several mechanisms including stimulation of tissue-specific G protein-coupled receptors. Vasopressin is non-selective, but its effects at the V1 receptor are responsible for the vasoconstrictor properties. Vasopressin blocks potassium-sensitive ATP channels, increasing smooth muscle intracellular calcium concentration, and improves vascular tone when noradrenaline receptor sensitivity is reduced. The dose range is 0.01 to 0.04 units/min. At higher doses, due to an increase in afterload, vasopressin increases myocardial oxygen demand and may induce myocardial ischaemia.

The Vasopressin in Septic Shock Trial (VASST) demonstrated a reduction in the amount of noradrenaline required, but showed no effect on mortality.

1.   Dellinger RP, Levy MM, Rhodes A, *et al*. Surviving Sepsis Campaign: international guidelines for management of severe sepsis and septic shock, 2012. *Intensive Care Med* 2013; 39(2): 165-228.
2.   Russell JA, Walley KR, Singer J, *et al*. Vasopressin versus norepinephrine infusion in patients with septic shock. *N Engl J Med* 2008; 358: 877-87.

5   F, F, F, T, T

Delirium is defined as a condition of altered consciousness, which develops acutely and shows a fluctuating clinical course. It is associated with increased length of stay, higher rates of nosocomial infection, decreased long-term cognitive function and increased mortality. Prevalence is high on the intensive care unit.

Subtypes include hyperactive, hypoactive and mixed. One prevalence study of medical ICU patients with delirium (Petersen *et al*) found that pure hyperactive (agitated) delirium was rare (around 2%), hypoactive common (43%), and mixed commonest (54%). Prophylaxis with haloperidol has recently been the subject of a randomised controlled trial within the UK, which failed to show a reduction in the incidence of delirium within the intervention group. The CAM-ICU assessment tool is a nationally adopted tool for delirium screening, which seeks to assess acuity of symptoms, inattention, altered level of consciousness and disorganised thinking. There is no test of recall or orientation.

Audiovisual reorientation has been suggested to be efficacious in the prevention and treatment of delirium. There are some RCT data to suggest that single-agent sedation with dexmedetomidine can reduce the incidence of delirium when compared to benzodiazepines, but there are limited data comparing against propofol, opiates and other modern sedative agents.

1. Reade MC, Finfer S. Sedation and delirium in the intensive care unit. *New Engl J Med* 2014; 370: 444-54.
2. Page VJ, Ely EW, Gates S, *et al*. Effect of intravenous haloperidol in the duration of delirium and coma in critically ill patients (Hope-ICU): a randomized, double blind, placebo controlled trial. *Lancet Respir Med* 2013; 1(7): 515-23.
3. Colombo R, Corona A, Praga F, *et al*. A reorientation strategy for reducing delirium in the critically ill. Results of an interventional study. *Minerva Anesthesiol* 2012; 78(9): 1026-33.
4. Riker RR, Shehabi Y, Bokesch PM, *et al*. Dexmedetomidine vs. midazolam for sedation of critically ill patients: a randomized trial. *JAMA* 2009; 301: 489-99.
5. Petersen JF, Pun BT, Dittus RS, *et al*. Delirium and its motoric subtypes: a study of 614 critically ill patients. *J Am Geriatric Soc* 2006; 54: 479-84.

6 F, F, T, F, T

The thyroid cartilage is situated at the level of C4-C5. The cricoid cartilage is situated at the level of C6. The cricothyroid membrane joins the cricoid and thyroid cartilages and is the preferred site for cricothyrotomy. On the right side the recurrent laryngeal nerve leaves the vagus as it crosses the subclavian artery, loops under the subclavian artery and ascends in the tracheo-oesophageal groove. On the left side it leaves the vagus as it crosses the aortic arch, loops under the arch and ascends in the tracheo-oesophageal groove. This puts the left recurrent laryngeal nerve at risk of damage from tumours of the lung, oesophagus and lymph nodes, as well as aortic aneurysms and an enlarged left atrium. The adult trachea is 15cm long. The window is opened for formal tracheostomy between the second and fourth tracheal rings. Any deviation from the midline increases the risk of vascular damage, including the anterior jugular vein, thyroidea ima artery, internal jugular vein and common carotid artery.

1.   Erdmann AG. *Concise Anatomy for Anaesthesia*. London, UK: Greenwich Medical Media, 2004.

7   T, T, F, T, F

Diabetic ketoacidosis management involves careful fluid and electrolyte management. Hypoglycaemia is common and may be as a result of insulin over-replacement. Serum phosphate often falls during treatment mainly as a result of intracellular shifts of potassium. This requires daily monitoring and appropriate replacement. Serum magnesium may also fall during insulin treatment.

Cerebral oedema mainly occurs in children but can also occur in adult patients and is often the result of rapid shifts in plasma osmolality. This can present as drowsiness, confusion and headaches. Such patients require HDU or ICU admission for observation and a low threshold for CT brain scan if the diagnosis is suspected.

Hyperchloraemic acidosis (with a high anion gap) may occur as a consequence of excessive saline infusions and increased bicarbonate consumption.

As a result of dehydration and tissue hypoperfusion, the risk of thromboembolism is increased and such cases require low-molecular-weight heparin for thromboprophylaxis.

1.   Joint British Diabetes Societies Inpatient Care Group. The management of diabetic ketoacidosis in adults, 2nd ed. London, UK: Joint British Diabetes Societies Inpatient Care Group for NHS Diabetes, 2013.
2.   Ramrakha PS, Moore KP, Sam A. Diabetic emergencies. *Oxford Handbook of Acute Medicine*, 3rd ed. Oxford, UK: Oxford University Press, 2010.

8   T, T, T, T, F

The anion gap can be calculated using the formula $(Na^+ + K^+) - (Cl^- + HCO_3)$. It has limitations, but remains useful when considering the underlying aetiology of an undifferentiated metabolic acidosis. An acidosis in this context can subsequently be divided into a high anion gap (HAGMA), a normal anion gap (NAGMA) and a low anion gap, which can help to rationalise further diagnostic testing. A normal anion gap is generally regarded as 8-16mEq/L, but this is dependent on the reference range used by the laboratory analysing the samples.

A normal anion gap acidosis is classically the result of a loss of base, but can also arise from exogenous administration of chloride-containing solutions.

A ureteroenterostomy leads to diversion of urine to the gut, for example, where urine with a high chloride load is reabsorbed resulting in excretion of bicarbonate and resultant hyperchloraemic metabolic acidosis. The same follows with exogenous administration of excess normal saline (although the resultant acid-base disturbance in this case may be better explained by Stewart's theory of strong ion difference). Addison's disease and carbonic anhydrase inhibitors are additional causes of a normal anion gap acidosis.

Diabetic ketoacidosis, lactic acidosis and poisoning with toxic alcohols or salicylates, all result in a raised anion gap metabolic acidosis.

1.   Kraut JA, Madias NE. Serum anion gap: its uses and limitations in clinical medicine. *Clin J Am Soc Nephrol* 2007; 2(1): 162-74.
2.   Badr A, Nightingale P. An alternative approach to acid-base abnormalities in critically ill patients. *Contin Educ Anaesth Crit Care Pain* 2007; 7(4): 107-11.

9   T, T, F, T, T

The common carotid artery ascends within the carotid sheath to divide (opposite the upper border of the thyroid cartilage — C4) into the internal and external carotid arteries. Three arteries supply the bowel: the coeliac trunk (supplies the stomach to the second part of the duodenum), the superior mesenteric artery (distal half of the second part of the duodenum to the junction of the proximal two thirds and distal third of the transverse colon) and the inferior mesenteric artery (distal third of the transverse colon to the rectum). Thus, disruption of the superior mesenteric artery is likely to cause ischaemia of the ileum. The great saphenous vein passes from the medial aspect of the foot, in front of the medial malleolus and then ascends on the medial side of the lower leg to the knee. Saphenous vein cut-down for intravenous access is performed where the vein passes anterior to the medial malleolus.

1.   Erdmann AG. *Concise Anatomy for Anaesthesia*. London, UK: Greenwich Medical Media, 2004.

10   F, F, T, F, T

The QT interval is defined as the period between the start of the QRS and the end of the T-wave. The corrected QT interval is calculated by the Bazzet's formula:

QTc = Q-T interval/square root of R-R interval

Common causes of long QT syndrome (LQTS) include: electrolyte disturbances (hypocalcaemia, hypokalaemia and low serum magnesium levels); medications (tricyclic antidepressants, antiarrhythmics such as amiodarone, phenothiazines, haloperidol); cardiac ischaemia;

subarachnoid haemorrhage; hypothermia; and congenital causes such as the Romano-Ward syndrome.

The main risk of LQTS is progression into the malignant torsades de points arrhythmia which requires emergency administration of intravenous magnesium and occasionally DC cardioversion. β-blockers reduce the incidence of arrhythmia in patients with LQTS through their adrenergic-blocking effect.

1. Viskin S. The QT interval: too long, too short or just right. *Heart Rhythm* 2009; 6(5): 711-5.
2. Wagner GS. *Marriott's Practical Electrocardiography*, 11th ed. Lippincott Williams & Wilkins, 2007.

11 F, F, F, F, F

The SAFE (Saline versus Albumin Fluid Evaluation) study investigators demonstrated no overt difference in outcomes between 7000 prospectively randomised, critically ill patients resuscitated with either 4.5% human albumin solution (HAS), or normal saline solution. However, in a subgroup analysis there was suggestion of worse outcomes for patients with traumatic brain injury receiving HAS, with an increased relative risk of death at 1.62 (95% confidence interval 1.12-2.35, p=0.009). This mortality increase persisted up to a year post-injury and was further analysed in a later paper. Despite this, the Lund protocol advocates the use of HAS in the management of traumatic brain injury as part of a strategy aiming to preserve capillary oncotic pressure to reduce cerebral oedema. This has not shown to be of benefit in randomised controlled trials, however.

Hydroxyethyl starch has recently been suspended by the Medicines and Healthcare Products Regulatory Agency (MHRA) regarding concerns of an increased incidence of acute kidney injury. These concerns have been highlighted in several systematic reviews. The risk of increased mortality is tenuous and dependent on study inclusion/assessment of bias within the reviews themselves. The use of hydroxyethyl starch 6% was shown to significantly increase mortality at 90 days in patients with severe sepsis when compared with balanced salt solution in the recent well-designed 6S trial.

The FEAST (Fluid Expansion As Supportive Therapy) trial noted a significantly increased mortality in critically ill children receiving a fluid bolus at 20-40ml/kg when compared to controls (no bolus).

1.   Finfer S, Bellomo R, Boyce N. The SAFE study investigators. A comparison of albumin and saline for fluid resuscitation in the intensive care unit. *New Engl J Med* 2004; 350(22): 2247-56.

2.   Finfer S, Bellomo R, Boyce N. The SAFE study investigators. Saline or albumin for fluid resuscitation in patients with traumatic brain injury. *New Engl J Med* 2007; 357: 874-84.

3.   Mutter TC, Ruth CA, Dart AB. Hydroxyethyl starch versus other fluid therapies: effects on kidney function. *Cochrane Database Syst Rev* 2013; 23: 7.

4.   Zarychanski R, Turgeon AF, Fergusson DA, *et al.* Association of hydroxyethyl starch administration with mortality and acute kidney injury in critically ill patients requiring volume resuscitation. *JAMA* 2013; 309(7): 678-88.

5.   Maitland K, Kiguli S, Opoka RO, *et al.* Mortality after fluid bolus in African children with severe infection *New Engl J Med* 2011; 364: 2483-95.

6.   Eker C, Asgeirsson B, Grände PO, *et al.* Improved outcome after severe head injury with a new therapy based on principles for brain volume regulation and preserved microcirculation. *Crit Care Med* 1998; 26: 1881-6.

7.   Perner A, Haase N, Guttormsen AB, *et al.* Hydroxyethyl starch 130/0.42 versus Ringer's acetate in severe sepsis. *N Engl J Med* 2012; 367: 124-34.

12   T, F, T, F, T

The spinal cord ends, on average, between L1 and L2 in the adult. Cerebrospinal fluid (CSF) is produced by the choroid plexuses of the lateral, third and fourth ventricles. It passes from the lateral ventricles to the third ventricle, then into the fourth ventricle. It then flows into the subarachnoid space. CSF is absorbed via the arachnoid villi and via lymphatic drainage. CSF pressure is gravitational. When lying, the opening CSF pressure is 6-10cm of CSF. In the sitting position, CSF pressure in the cervical region is sub-atmospheric and 20-40cm of CSF in the lumbar area.

1.   Erdmann AG. *Concise Anatomy for Anaesthesia.* London, UK: Greenwich Medical Media, 2004.

13 T, F, T, T, F

The arterial waveform results from ejection of blood from the left ventricle into the aorta during systole, followed by peripheral arterial flow of this stroke volume during diastole. The area under the systolic portion of the waveform up to the dicrotic notch represents the stroke volume. The dicrotic notch represents the closure of the aortic valve. The dP/dt is an index of contractility. Important impressions of volume state can be made from the arterial waveform and its characteristics, for example, a vasodilated circulation is indicated by a steep diastolic rate of decay while a hypovolaemic state is suggested by an arterial waveform with a low dicrotic notch and a narrow waveform. The 'delta down' is a measure of the reduction in arterial systolic pressure from baseline (measured at end-expiratory pause) during mechanical ventilation, and reflects the normal decrease in venous return during inspiration. It is greater in magnitude in patients who are hypovolaemic.

1. Yentis SM. Hirsch NP, Smith GB. *Anaesthesia and Intensive Care A-Z*, 3rd ed. London, UK: Butterworth-Heinemann, 2004.
2. Perel A, Pizov R, Cotev V. Systolic pressure variation is a sensitive indicator of hypovolaemia in ventilated dogs subjected to graded haemorrhage. *Anaesthesiology* 1987; 67: 498-502.

14 F, F, F, T, T

The pulmonary artery catheter is now a relatively infrequent tool within the intensive care unit, following suggestions of limited benefit from randomised controlled trials alongside a significant risk profile. However, they are still used in challenging clinical situations and an understanding of insertion technique, calibration, thermodilution and interpretation remains important to the practising critical care physician.

Insertion of the catheter can lead to direct measurement of multiple variables, including central venous pressure, right atrial pressure, right ventricular systolic pressure, pulmonary artery pressure, and pulmonary artery occlusion pressure (a surrogate for left atrial pressure, although it should be noted that this is not directly measured *per se*) and mixed venous oxygen saturations.

This information, along with central thermodilution and additional measurements, can lead to assessment and calculation of multiple indirect variables, including cardiac output, cardiac index, oxygen delivery, systemic vascular resistance and pulmonary vascular resistance.

1.   Reade MC, Angus DC. PAC-Man: game over for the pulmonary artery catheter? *Crit Care* 2006; 10: 303.

15   T, F, F, T, T

Many drugs exert their effects by binding to a receptor. Receptors are generally protein or glycoprotein in nature and may lie in the cell membrane, cytosol or the cell nucleus. Receptors can be categorised according to the effect an agonist causes: alteration in ion permeability, production of intermediate messengers and regulation of gene transcription. Ligand binding can alter the permeability of the ion channel to ions. The nicotinic receptor at the neuromuscular junction is a ligand gated ion channel and is the site of action of suxamethonium. G proteins are a complex series of proteins which act via the production of intermediate messengers. Stimulation of Gs proteins activates adenylate cyclase, thus increasing the production of cyclic adenosine monophosphate (cAMP). Stimulation of Gi proteins inhibits adenylate cyclase, thus decreasing the production of cAMP. Activation of Gt proteins activates guanylate cyclase which catalyses the formation of cyclic guanosine monophosphate (cGMP). Ligands at Gt proteins include atrial natriuretic peptide and nitric oxide. Gq proteins are activated by ligand binding; this activates phospholipase C which breaks down phosphoinositol (a membrane phospholipid) into second messengers. α1-adrenoceptors and angiotensin I exert their effects via Gq proteins. Tyrosine kinase is contained within the cell membrane and activated by certain drugs and natural compounds controlling cell growth and differentiation by regulation of gene transcription. Insulin and growth factor work via the tyrosine kinase system. Steroids and thyroid hormones act to alter the expression of DNA and RNA within the cytosol and cell nucleus.

1. Peck TE, Williams M. *Pharmacology for Anaesthesia and Intensive Care*. London, UK: Greenwich Medical Media, 2002.

16 F, T, F, T, T

One requirement for continuous renal replacement therapy (CRRT) including haemofiltration is the need for anticoagulation. This may increase the likelihood for bleeding in the patient. However, in the absence of effective anticoagulation, this may result in clotting of the filter and inefficient renal replacement therapy. Blood flow, dialyser type, coagulation pathway activation, and convective mass transfer are among the factors which may increase the risk of clotting problems. Heparins are widely used for anticoagulation, but due to their potential side effects such as bleeding and heparin-induced thrombocytopaenia, alternative anticoagulation protocols should be considered. These include citrate anticoagulation, regional heparin/protamine, pre-dilution, and prostacyclin.

Regional citrate use in the extracorporeal circuit provides anticoagulation by chelating calcium, and calcium is necessary for blood coagulation. This effect is reversed by calcium infusion into the systemic circulation. Citrate metabolism in liver and skeletal muscle generates bicarbonate. Hypernatraemia, metabolic alkalosis, hypocalcaemia, and hypercalcaemia are potential complications of this anticoagulation method.

Increasing the proportion of replacement fluid delivered pre-filter (predilution) will decrease the viscosity of blood in the circuit and decrease clotting risk at the expense of less efficient clearance of solutes. Drugs such as prostacyclin (epoprostenol) that inhibit interaction between platelets and artificial membranes were introduced as an alternative anticoagulant strategy for CRRT.

1. Schetz, M. Anticoagulation for continuous renal replacement therapy. *Curr Opin Anaesthesiol* 2001; 14: 143-9.
2. http://www.kdigo.org/clinical_practice_guidelines/pdf/KDIGO%20AKI%20Guideline.pdf (accessed 12th September 2014).

17   T, F, T, F, T

The oesophageal Doppler cardiac output monitor uses the Doppler principle to measure the velocity time integral for blood flow in the descending aorta. Coupled to an estimation of aortic root cross-sectional area and mathematical modelling, these data can produce estimates of stroke volume and cardiac output via a minimally invasive means.

Oesophageal Doppler monitoring works under two key assumptions. Firstly, that derivation of aortic cross-sectional area is estimated — this is usually via a specific nomogram. Secondly, that a constant percentage of the cardiac output enters the descending aorta, as measurements with the probe clearly exclude coronary and cerebral circulations. As such, a correction factor must be applied to the readings to give true cardiac output.

Peak velocity is an age-dependent measure of contractility, independent of afterload. The flow time (FT) is dependent on heart rate, and as such is usually corrected using a derivation of Bazett's formula to a rate of 60bpm (1 second per cardiac cycle). As such, systolic flow time should be roughly a third of this and so a normal FTc has a range of 330 to 360 milliseconds. A high FTc usually reflects a reduction in afterload such that the systolic time promotes extended flow. This can be seen in vasoplegia from sepsis and drug administration, but should be balanced against the shortening of the FTc that can be seen with either preload reduction or occasionally, myocardial depression.

There are multiple relative contraindications to insertion, including nasal trauma, oesophageal varices, surgery, stent or carcinoma, and intra-aortic balloon pump placement. While the probe is commonly placed via the nasal route, it can be passed orally into the oesophagus in cases of nasal injury or suspected base of skull fracture.

1.   King SL, Lim MS. The use of the oesophageal Doppler monitor in the intensive care unit. *Crit Care Resusc* 2004; 6: 113-22.
2.   Singer M. Oesophageal Doppler. *Curr Opin Crit Care* 2009; 15: 244-8.

18 F, F, T, F, F

A creatinine clearance of 30-59ml/min denotes moderate renal impairment (chronic kidney disease stage 3). Many renally excreted drugs need dose adjustment to prevent accumulation of the drug with potentially serious side effects (Table 2.1).

Table 2.1. Examples of dose adjustments for common antimicrobials in the presence of renal impairment.

Drug	Route	Normal dosing schedule	Moderate renal impairment CrCl 30-59ml/min	Severe renal impairment CrCl 10-29ml/min	Very severe renal impairment CrCl <10ml/min
Amphotericin B lipid preparation	IV	3-5mg/kg Q24h	No change	No change	No change
Clarithromycin	IV/PO	500mg Q12h	No change	No change	No change
Meropenem	IV	1-2g Q8h	1-2g bd	1g bd or 500mg tds	1-2g od
Metronidazole	IV	500mg Q8h	No change	No change	No change
	PO	400mg Q8h	No change	No change	No change
Tazocin	IV	4.5g Q8h-Q6h	No change	CrCl 10-20ml/min 4.5g Q12h	4.5g Q12h

1. Ashley C, Currie A, Eds. *The Renal Drug Handbook*, 3rd ed. London, UK: Radcliffe Publishing, 2004.

19 T, F, F, F, T

About 20-25% (range 17-40%) of the 150,000 ischaemic strokes in the United Kingdom each year affect posterior circulation brain structures (including the brainstem, cerebellum, midbrain, thalamus, and areas of temporal and occipital cortex), which are supplied by the vertebrobasilar arterial system and therefore not assessed by routine carotid Doppler assessment. Early recognition of posterior circulation stroke or transient ischaemic attack (TIA) may prevent disability and save lives; however, it remains more difficult to recognise and treat effectively than other stroke types. Delayed or incorrect diagnosis may have devastating consequences, including potentially preventable death or severe disability. Preceding posterior circulation TIA or other transient brainstem symptoms, particularly if recurrent, signal a high risk of impending ischaemic stroke and should prompt urgent specialist referral. Such posterior circulation strokes may lead to oedema and swelling in areas of the brain with limited capacity for expansion, thus leading to the need for neurosurgical decompression procedures. The risk of recurrent stroke after posterior circulation stroke is at least as high as for anterior circulation stroke, and vertebrobasilar stenosis increases the risk three-fold.

1.   Merwick Á, Werring D. Posterior circulation ischaemic stroke. *Br Med J* 2014; 348: g3175.

20   T, F, F, F, F

The intra-aortic balloon pump (IABP) is one of the most widely used circulatory assist devices for critically ill patients. Although supporting evidence is limited, it remains a regularly utilised therapy and as such the practising intensivist must understand the principles and rationale for insertion.

The primary role of the IABP is to increase myocardial oxygen supply and thus facilitate an improvement in ventricular performance. It achieves this by inflating at the onset of diastole, timed with the dichrotic notch, to increase coronary perfusion pressure prior to the next systolic contraction. The balloon deflates just before systole, thus reducing afterload and further improving cardiac performance. Proposed indications for insertion include acute myocardial infarction, cardiogenic shock, ventricular failure and cardiac surgery.

Helium is used to inflate the balloon to provide rapid gas transfer via laminar flow and to allow absorption within the bloodstream in the unlikely event of balloon rupture. The balloon is positioned 2-3cm distal to the origin of the left subclavian artery.

Trial data supporting use are weak. A systematic review has suggested insufficient evidence to support incorporation to guidelines. In 2012, the further results of IABP Shock II suggested no difference in mortality for patients with acute myocardial infarction complicated by cardiogenic shock randomised to IABP or conservative management.

1. Krishna M, Zacharowski K. Principles of intra-aortic balloon pump counterpulsation. *Contin Educ Anaesth Crit Care Pain* 2009; 9(1): 24-8.
2. Sjauw KD, Engström AE, Vis MM, *et al*. A systematic review and meta-analysis of intra-aortic balloon pump therapy in ST-elevation myocardial infarction: should we change the guidelines? *Eur Heart J* 2009; 30(4): 459-68.
3. Thiele H, Zeymer U, Neumann FJ, *et al*. Intra-aortic balloon support for myocardial infarction with cardiogenic shock *New Engl J Med* 2012; 367(14): 1287-96.

21 T, T, F, T, F

pH, PCO_2 and PO_2 are direct measurements and HCO_3^-, base excess and oxygen saturations are derived measurements. The electrodes in the blood gas analyser are maintained within narrow limits (37+/- 0.1°C) and the blood sample is warmed to this value before it is analysed. pH, and PCO_2 and PO_2 change with a change in temperature. Blood gas machines can calculate a pH, PCO_2 and PO_2 value for the actual patient temperature. Gas is less soluble (and therefore has a higher partial pressure) at higher temperatures in the bloodstream, therefore a blood sample from a hypothermic patient analysed at 37°C will overestimate the true $PaCO_2$ or PaO_2. Depending on the concentration gradient between the blood sample and air bubbles, oxygen will diffuse into or out of the blood sample leading to either an increase or decrease in the measured PO_2. In extreme leukocytosis, oxygen consumption occurs and pseudohypoxaemia is seen.

1. Nickson C. Arterial blood gas in hypothermia. Life in the fast lane. http://lifeinthefastlane.com/education/ccc/arterial-blood-gas-in-hypothermia (accessed 3rd August 2014).
2. Bersten AD, Soni N. *Oh's Intensive Care Manual*, 6th ed. Philadelphia, USA: Butterworth Heinemann, Elsevier, 2009.

22 F, F, T, T, T

Normal intracranial pressure is between 5 and 15mmHg. There are rhythmic variations in ICP, named Lundberg A, B and C pressure waves. Although B and C waves are associated with variations of respiratory movements and blood pressure, A (or plateau) waves are sustained elevations of intracranial pressure lasting for several minutes. They signify raised intracranial pressure. Sneezing, coughing and straining can increase ICP by 45mmHg.

Normal ICP waveforms are similar to the arterial waveform, with a first peak (P1, percussion wave) correlating with systole, a second peak (P2, dicrotic wave) which correlates with aortic valve closure, and a third peak (P3, tidal wave) correlating with antegrade arterial flow during diastole; as intracranial compliance falls, the morphology of the ICP waveform also changes, with the amplitude of the dicrotic wave, the second peak, initially equals and then exceeds the amplitude of the percussion wave.

The primary goal of ICP management is to maintain ICP below 20mmHg and cerebral perfusion pressure (CPP) above 60mmHg. While elimination of the cause of elevated ICP remains the definitive approach, there are interventions that should be used to decrease ICP urgently, while CPP management should be emphasised.

1.   Sabdoughi A, Rybinnik I, Cohen R. Measurement and management of increased intracranial pressure. *Crit Care Med J* 2013; 6 (Suppl 1: M4): 56-65.

23 T, T, F, F, F

Weaning from mechanical ventilation is the stepwise process of reducing respiratory support with the ultimate aim of extubation and satisfactory spontaneous breathing. Many critically ill patients will tolerate this process rapidly following improvement from their acute event. Some patients will need a more gradual approach.

General features associated with successful weaning include improvement in the underlying condition, optimisation of general physiology and identification of potentially deleterious airway or breathing issues. Following this, numerical indices are a fairly reliable way of predicting the likelihood of success with a spontaneous breathing trial and have been consistently shown to outperform clinical judgement when used systematically.

Numerical indices in current use include the Rapid Shallow Breathing Index <105 (respiratory rate divided by tidal volume measured in litres), respiratory rate in isolation (<35/min), vital capacity >10ml/kg and PaO_2/FiO_2 >26kPa. However, there remain concerns regarding the sensitivity and specificity of chosen cut-offs and they must be used as part of a rational decision-making process, rather than as standalone targets. Isolated measurements of PO_2 or CO_2 have a limited role.

1.   Lermitte J, Garfield MJ. Weaning from mechanical ventilation. *Contin Educ Anaesth Crit Care Pain* 2005; 5: 113-7.

24   F, F, F, F, T

The Sengstaken-Blakemore tube is used in the temporary management of bleeding varices. It can be inserted orally or nasally and can be used in awake patients. The tube has oesophageal and gastric balloons and one port to aspirate gastric contents. The Minnesota tube has an additional port to aspirate oesophageal contents in an attempt to reduce the risk of aspiration pneumonia. The tube is inserted to the 55cm mark (indicating a position well below the gastro-oesophageal junction), the gastric balloon inflated with water or air, and the position checked with radiography. Once the position is confirmed the gastric balloon is completely inflated. The tube is then pulled back until resistance is felt. If bleeding continues, the oesophageal balloon can also be insufflated. Weighted traction using bags of saline is no longer recommended as it can lead to necrosis at the gastro-oesophageal junction and at the angle of the mouth. Traction on the tube is best applied using tape to the skin of the nose only. The use of a

Sengstaken-Blakemore tube is associated with serious complications such as oesophageal ulceration, oesophageal perforation and aspiration pneumonia in 15-20% of cases. Up to 50% of patients will rebleed once the balloon is deflated, so its primary function is to control bleeding prior to further definitive treatment.

1.   Waldmann C, Soni N, Rhodes A. *Oxford Desk Reference Critical Care*. Oxford, UK: Oxford University Press, 2008.

25   F, F, F, T, T

Among the common associated risk factors for development of acute kidney injury in the postoperative period are: pre-existing renal insufficiency; Type 1 diabetes mellitus; patient age over 65 years; major vascular surgery; cardiopulmonary bypass times over 3 hours; and recent exposure to nephrotoxic agents (such as radio-contrast dyes, bile pigments, aminoglycoside, antibiotics, and NSAIDs).

1.   Sear JW. Kidney dysfunction in the postoperative period. *Br J Anaesth* 2005; 95(1): 20-32.

26   T, T, T, F, F

Continuous positive airway pressure has multiple physiological ramifications within the intensive care unit. While it may be a very familiar treatment, understanding of these effects will lead to best use in clinical practice.

Functional residual capacity (FRC) will impact on gas transfer due to an impact on alveolar surface area available for exchange. Positive end-expiratory pressure (PEEP) can reduce atelectasis and maintain recruitment of collapsed alveoli, thus increasing the FRC and subsequently increasing surface area for the transfer of oxygen to the bloodstream.

PEEP can also have important cardiovascular effects such as a reduction in preload, redistribution of extravascular lung water (secondary to increased hydrostatic pressure within the alveoli) and decreased left ventricular afterload. This latter feature has led some authors to suggest that PEEP can increase cardiac output, although the general consensus at present suggests that the impact of decreased preload and consequent decreased left ventricular filling cause little positive effect on cardiac output. In a small cohort of patients with a failing myocardium and hypervolaemia (congestive cardiac failure), PEEP may result in improved cardiac output due to the decrease in afterload providing greater overall benefit. There is trial evidence to support CPAP in this situation to reduce symptoms and work of breathing.

PEEP will invariably increase intracranial pressure by impairing venous drainage to the thorax, resulting in a degree of intracranial venous congestion and resultant pressure increase alongside volume expansion.

1. Luecke T, Pelosi P. Clinical review: positive end-expiratory pressure and cardiac output. *Crit Care* 2005; 9(6): 607-21.
2. Gray A, Goodacre S, Newby DE, *et al*. Non-invasive ventilation in acute cardiogenic pulmonary oedema. *New Engl J Med* 2008; 359: 142-51.

27 T, F, F, T, F

The neurological level of a spinal cord injury is defined as the lowest level of the spinal cord with normal sensation and motor function on both sides of the body. Due to secondary injury, cord ischaemia extends bi-directionally from the site of injury over the first 72 hours which may manifest as an ascending neurological level and lead to clinical deterioration. Spinal cord injuries above the level of T8 lead to impaired ventilation due to a loss of inspiratory intercostal and abdominal muscles. If the injury is between C3-5, there is partial phrenic nerve denervation and above C3, total diaphragmatic paralysis occurs. In a high spinal cord injury, lying flat improves respiratory function as the diaphragm has a greater excursion in inspiration as it is pushed into the chest by the abdominal contents. Gastroparesis may occur due to unopposed vagal activity. Feeding patients with high cord lesions enterally may lead to vomiting, abdominal distension and the risk of aspiration; however, early enteral feeding has been shown to decrease mortality in polytrauma patients and enteral feed should be attempted within the first 24 hours after injury. Rates of deep vein thrombosis (DVT) are as stated. Intermittent calf compression devices or graduated compression stockings should be used as prophylaxis for DVT during the first 48-72 hours because of the risk of bleeding around the cord. After 72 hours, prophylactic low-molecular-weight heparin should be commenced, unless contraindicated due to other injuries. Acute denervation of the motor end plate leads to spread of acetylcholine receptors beyond the motor end plate and after 72 hours the use of suxamethonium may precipitate life-threatening hyperkalaemia. This effect resolves after approximately 6 months and suxamethonium can again be safely used.

1.   Bonner S, Smith C. Initial management of acute spinal cord injury. *Contin Educ Anaesth Crit Care Pain* 2013; 13(6): 224-31.

28   F, F, F, T, F

The acute management of Wolff-Parkinson-White (WPW) syndrome with tachycardia is divided into the following:

- Unstable: synchronised DC shock.
- Stable: anti-arrhythmic agents which cause prolongation of the accessory pathway such as sotalol, procainamide, flecainide and amiodarone.

There are important differences between the pathophysiology of regular narrow complex tachyarrhythmias in this condition compared with the tachyarrhythmia of atrial fibrillation (AF) with rapid ventricular response and this has implications for the drugs used to terminate acute episodes.

In the case of atrioventricular reentrant tachycardias (AVRT) or AV nodal reentrant tachycardias (AVNRT), AV node-blocking drugs such as adenosine and verapamil can be used to break the cycle of reentrant electrical activity. However, the use of AV node-blocking drugs in atrial fibrillation with fast ventricular response is contraindicated, as in this situation atrial electrical activity will be conducted with greater frequency to the ventricles via the accessory pathway (since the AV node is blocked), risking increased ventricular rate and deterioration into a malignant rhythm.

β-blockers, digoxin, adenosine and verapamil all have a blocking action on the AV node and hence should be avoided. Amiodarone may also have a similar action and should be avoided in this situation also. Suitable agents include Class Ic drugs such as flecainide and propafenone, and Class III agents such as ibutilide.

The management and diagnosis of tachyarrhythmias in WPW syndrome is complex and expert advice should be sought if the patient is haemodynamically stable.

1. Di Biase L, Walsh EP. Treatment of symptomatic arrhythmias associated with the Wolff-Parkinson-White syndrome, 2014. *UpToDate*. http://www.uptodate.com/contents/treatment-of-symptomatic-arrhythmias-associated-with-the-wolff-parkinson-white-syndrome (accessed January 2nd 2015).

29   F, F, T, F, T

Major burns are associated with a significant incidence of death and disability, multiple surgical procedures, prolonged hospital stay and organ support. Critical care must be fastidious and aggressive. A recent Cochrane review assessing the use of antibiotic therapy to reduce the risk of burn wound infection found no benefit to the use of selective digestive tract decontamination (SDD). In fact, a statistically significant increase in the development of methicillin-resistant *Staphylococcus aureus* (MRSA) was noted.

Initial treatment consists of fluid replacement, wound care and organ support. Fluid prescription is still guided by the Parkland formula in the early stages of care, which suggests 3-4ml/kg/% TBSA burn over the first 24-hour period, with any prehospital fluid subtracted from the total, and the first half given over the first 8 hours. When calculating total body surface area, erythematous regions are omitted unless there is additional blistering or underlying evidence of partial-thickness burns.

The Baux score approximates mortality risk using the formula: age of patient + percentage TBSA burned. A modified score has also been proposed adding an additional 17% for airway burns involvement.

1.   Barajas-Nava LA, López-Alcalde J, Roqué i Figuls M, *et al*. Antibiotic prophylaxis for preventing burn wound infection. *Cochrane Database Syst Rev* 2013; 6: CD008738.
2.   Benson A, Dickson WA, Boyce DE. ABC of wound healing: burns. *Br Med J* 2006; 332: 649.
3.   Roberts G, Lloyd M, Parker M, *et al*. The Baux score is dead. Long live the Baux score. A 27-year retrospective cohort study of mortality at a regional burns service. *J Trauma Acute Care Surg* 2012; 72(1): 251-6.

30   F, T, F, F, F

The FAST (Face, Arm, Speech, Time to call 999) test is publicised in the UK to diagnose stroke. It has a positive predictive value of approximately 80%. The ROSIER (Recognition of Stroke in the Emergency Room) scale for stroke assessment enables medical staff to differentiate between patients with stroke and stroke mimics. It has a sensitivity of 93%. ABCD (Age, Blood pressure, Clinical features, Duration and Diabetes) is used in patients who have had a suspected TIA to assess their 7-day risk of developing a stroke. The National Institutes of Health Stroke Scale is used to quantify the impairment caused by a stroke. Eleven items are scored and total scores range from 0 (no stroke) to 42 (severe stroke). UK expert consensus does not currently recommend the routine use of prophylactic low-molecular-weight heparin in addition to full-dose aspirin, or the immediate commencement of statin treatment due to the risk of haemorrhagic transformation. Patients already taking statins should continue this therapy, as there is clear long-term benefit. All patients should be considered for statin therapy after 48 hours although immediate statin therapy is not currently recommended in consensus guidelines. There is evidence from three small European randomised controlled trials (DECIMAL [Decompressive Craniectomy In Malignant Middle Cerebral Artery Infarcts], DESTINY [DEcompressive Surgery for the Treatment of malignant INfarction of the middle cerebral arterY] and HAMLET [Hemicraniectomy After Middle cerebral artery infarction with Life-threatening Edema Trial]) that decompressive hemicraniectomy is potentially life-saving in patients with malignant middle cerebral artery infarction. These trials enrolled patients aged 18-60 years and there is currently no evidence to support the use of decompressive craniectomy in patients >60 years of age.

1. Raithatha A, Pratt G, Rash A. Developments in the management of acute ischaemic stroke: implications for anaesthetic and critical care management. *Contin Educ Anaesth Crit Care Pain* 2013; 13(3): 80-6.
2. Royal College of Physicians. Diagnosis and initial management of transient ischaemic attack. London, UK: RCP, 2010.
3. National Institute for Health and Clinical Excellence. Stroke: diagnosis and initial management of acute stroke and transient ischaemic attack (TIA). NICE clinical guideline 68. London, UK: NICE, 2008. www.nice.org.uk (accessed 25th February 2015).
4. Vahedi K, Hofmeijer J, Juettler E, *et al*, for the DECIMAL, DESTINY, and HAMLET investigators. Early decompressive surgery in malignant infarction of the middle cerebral artery: a pooled analysis of three randomized controlled trials. *Lancet Neurol* 2007; 6: 315-22.

31 T, T, F, F, T

Amitriptyline overdose effects are mainly due to anticholinergic (atropine-like) effects at autonomic nerve endings and in the brain. Peripheral symptoms therefore include sinus tachycardia, hot dry skin, dry mouth and tongue, dilated pupils and urinary retention. The most important electrocardiographic (ECG) feature of toxicity is prolongation of the QRS interval, which indicates a high risk of progression to ventricular tachycardia and other malignant arrhythmias including Torsades de pointes.

Tachyarrhythmias are most appropriately treated by correction of hypoxia and acidosis. Patients with prolongation of the QRS complex, hypotension or tachyarrhythmias should be treated with intravenous sodium bicarbonate even in the absence of acidosis. Alkalinisaton promotes dissociation of the tricyclic drug from myocardial sodium channels and therefore reduces its cardiotoxic effects.

Neurological features of severe tricyclic poisoning include ataxia, nystagmus and drowsiness, which may lead to deep coma and respiratory depression. There may be increased tone and hyperreflexia together with extensor plantar reflexes. Seizures may occur and are best treated by supportive care and administration of intravenous benzodiazepines. Phenytoin is contraindicated in tricyclic overdose, because, like tricyclic antidepressants, it blocks sodium channels and may increase the risk of cardiac arrhythmias. Glucagon has been used to correct myocardial depression and hypotension.

1. Katzung B, Masters S, Trevor A. *Basic and Clinical Pharmacology*, 11th ed. San Francisco, USA: McGraw-Hill, 2009.
2. MHRA. Regulating medicine and medicines devices. Amitriptyline overdose. http//www.mhra.gov.uk (accessed May 1st 2014).
3. Hoffman JR, Votey SR, Bayer M, Silver L. Effect of hypertonic sodium bicarbonate in the treatment of moderate-to-severe cyclic antidepressant overdose. *Am J Emerg Med* 1993; 11: 336-41.

32   T, T, F, T, F

The intentional nature of many ingestions coupled to the characteristics of this patient cohort unfortunately limit the availability of randomised controlled trial data. Management is usually based on pharmacological studies and expert advice, provided by the National Poisons Information Service. Recent review articles highlight specific developments and focus on critical care.

Ingestion of toxic alcohol is still frequently encountered and can lead to severe clinical sequelae. Treatment is via competitive inhibition of alcohol dehydrogenase using either ethanol or fomepizole. Cyanide poisoning can be managed with sodium thiosulphate, dicobalt edetate or hydroxycobalamin in the form of a cyanokit. Thiosulphate is a substrate which allows mitochondrial metabolism of cyanide to harmless thiocyanate. β-blockade overdose is notoriously troublesome to manage and often requires central venous access and ionotropic support. Large doses of intravenous glucagon are recommended initially and the use of high-dose insulin euglycaemic therapy (HIET) is gaining momentum following relative success in the treatment of calcium channel blocker overdose.

Organophosphate poisoning causes a cholinergic toxidrome which can be managed with atropine or pralidoxime. Pralidoxime causes displacement of the organophosphate from the acetylcholinesterase enzyme which the poison inhibits. Paraquat ingestion is worsened by oxygen, which worsens the extent of lung damage. Fuller's earth is a recognised treatment (although not a specific antidote).

1. Alapat PM, Zimmerman JL. Toxicology in the critical care unit. *Chest* 2008; 133: 1006-13.
2. Lheureux PER, Wood DM, Wright KD, *et al.* Bench to bedside review: hyperinsulinaemia/euglycaemia therapy in the management of overdose of calcium channel blockers. *Crit Care* 2006; 10: 212.

33 T, F, F, T, T

A quality-adjusted life-year (QALY) takes into account both the quantity and quality of life generated after healthcare interventions. A year of perfect health is worth 1. Death is considered to be equivalent to 0; however, some health states may be considered worse than death and have negative scores. The use of QALYs allows cost-utility ratios to be calculated for an intervention, allowing comparisons between interventions and allocation of resources.

The QALY is an objective measure of quality of life. Subjective measures commonly used in intensive care include the EuroQol-5D, SF-36 (Medical Outcomes Study 36-item Short-Form Health Survey), RAND-36 (RAND 36-Item Health Survey) and NHP (Nottingham Health Profile) tools. Subjective measures are more suited to the critical care population. EQ-5D is a short questionnaire with three parts. A descriptive system measures health in five domains: mobility, self-care, usual activities, pain/discomfort and anxiety/depression. Each domain has three levels: no problems, moderate problems or severe problems. Patients also rate their health between 0 and 100 using a visual analogue scale. The Hospital Anxiety and Depression Scale is a well-validated subjective measure of quality of life. It is a short questionnaire which takes 2-5 minutes to complete and, using questions regarding anxiety and depression, provides the medical practitioner with valuable information regarding the mental state of the patient. The SF-36 questionnaire contains 36 items measuring eight multi-item domains: physical and social functioning, role limitations caused by physical or emotional problems, mental health, vitality, bodily pain and general perception of health. The RAND-36 questionnaire was developed from the SF-36 and produces virtually identical results as the SF-36. The NHP consists of a two-part questionnaire. The first part has 38 statements related to six domains, the second part lists seven activities of daily life. The NHP has poorer consistency and sensitivity to change than the SF-36 and RAND-36.

1. Phillips C. What is a QALY? April 2009. http://www.medicine.ox.ac.uk/bandolier/painres/download/whatis/QALY.pdf (accessed 17th July 2014).
2. Bersten AD, Soni N. *Oh's Intensive Care Manual*, 6th ed. Philadelphia, USA: Butterworth Heinemann, Elsevier, 2009.
3. Oeyen SG, Vandijick DM, Benoit DD, *et al*. Quality of life after intensive care: a systematic review of the literature. *Crit Care Med* 2010; 38(12): 2386-400.
4. Snaith RP. The Hospital Anxiety and Depression Scale. *Health Qual Life Out* 2003; 1: 29.

34   F, T, T, T, F

Toxic shock syndrome (TSS) is caused by a bacterial exotoxin and is associated with a high mortality rate and risk of multi-organ dysfunction. Up to 90% of cases occur in females. Retained tampons are common causes, but around 50% of cases of TSS have an alternative cause such as surgical wound infections, burns, cutaneous lesions or osteomyelitis. TSS is caused by Gram-positive bacteria including *Staphylococcus aureus* and group A *Streptococci*.

For staphylococcal toxic shock syndrome, the diagnosis is based strictly upon Centers for Disease Control and Prevention (CDC) criteria defined in 2011, based on the presence of clinical and laboratory criteria.

There are five clinical criteria: fever; maculopapular rash; desquamation (1-2 weeks following rash); hypotension; and multisystem involvement (three of gastrointestinal, mucous membranes, muscular, renal, hepatic, haematological and central nervous system). Laboratory criteria are negative results of blood cultures (with the exception of a positive *S. aureus* blood culture) and negative serology for Rocky Mountain fever, leptospirosis and measles. Cases are considered to be confirmed if all diagnostic criteria are present (unless the patient dies before the desquamation process). A case is considered probable if four clinical criteria in addition to laboratory criteria are met.

Due to the potential high morbidity and mortality of the condition, patients are often most appropriately managed in an intensive care unit for fluid management and advanced organ support. Source control is of paramount importance including drainage of abscesses and collections, and removal of the retained tampon if this is the culprit. Treatment includes anti-staphylococcal antibiotics such as high-dose intravenous flucloxacillin or teicoplanin. Toxin production and mortality can also be reduced by the addition of clindamycin or gentamicin.

1. Toxic shock syndrome (other than streptococcal) (TSS): 2011 case definition. Centers for Disease Control and Prevention, May 8th 2014.
2. Zimbelman J, Palmer A, Todd J. Improved outcome of clindamycin compared with beta-lactam antibiotic treatment for invasive *Streptococcus pyogenes* infection. *Ped Infect Dis J* 1999; 18(12): 1096-100.
3. Venkataraman R, Pinsky MR. Toxic shock syndrome. http://emedicine.medscape.com/article/169177-overview (accessed 7th January 2015).

35   T, T, T, F, F

Upper gastrointestinal bleeding is a common reason for admission to an intensive care unit, requiring multidisciplinary liaison for definitive care alongside meticulous supportive therapy.

Recent RCT evidence is strongly suggestive of a reduction in mortality with a transfusion trigger of 70g/L, as well as a reduction in rebleeding, adverse events and portal pressure gradient. The use of antibiotics in cirrhotic patients has been shown to decrease the rate of serious bacterial infection and subsequent all cause mortality at systematic review. Terlipressin causes splanchnic vasoconstriction and thus promotes haemostasis at the site of variceal haemorrhage. A systematic review has previously demonstrated a mortality reduction when compared against placebo in patients with acute variceal bleeding.

Sengstaken-Blakemore and Minnesota tube placement offers balloon tamponade as a bridge to definitive treatment for variceal bleeding, such as TIPSS (transjugular intrahepatic portosystemic shunting). It is a rescue therapy based on expert opinion and has little to offer in the acute setting prior to endoscopy unless the patient is exsanguinating. There is scant evidence describing use and no randomised controlled trial data suggestive of benefit.

Current NICE guidance suggests avoiding prescription of proton pump inhibitors (PPIs) until endoscopy has been performed in order to accurately identify bleeding lesions and tailor therapy appropriately. This recommendation is based on the recent Cochrane review that suggested pre-endoscopy PPI medications to show no improvement in clinically important outcomes, such as mortality, rebleed rates or the need for surgery.

1.   Villanueva C, Colomo A, Bosch A, *et al.* Transfusion strategies for acute upper gastrointestinal bleeding. *New Engl J Med* 2013; 368: 11-21.
2.   Chavez-Tapia NC, Barrientos-Gutierrez T, Tellez-Avila F, *et al.* Antibiotic prophylaxis for cirrhotic patients with acute upper gastrointestinal bleeding. *Cochrane Database Syst Rev* 2010; 9: CD002907.
3.   Ioannou G, Doust J, Rockey DC. Systematic review: terlipressin in acute oesophageal haemorrhage. *Aliment Pharmacol Ther* 2003; 17: 53-64.
4.   Sreedharan A, Martin J, Leontiadis GI, *et al.* Proton pump inhibitor treatment initiated prior to endoscopic diagnosis in upper gastrointestinal bleeding. *Cochrane Database Syst Rev* 2010; 7: CD005415.

36   F, F, T, F, F

The vast majority of ICU patients lack the capacity to be involved in discussions regarding withholding or withdrawal of treatment. When patients are admitted to the ICU there should be a clear management plan encompassing the limits, if any, of invasive interventions. This plan requires regular (but not necessarily daily) review and updating. The decision to withdraw or withhold is normally taken after consultation with other members of the nursing and medical team. Unanimity is desirable but may be unobtainable. The final decision, and responsibility for the decision, is vested in the consultant in charge of the ICU, but it is essential that the views of the family, or those close to the patient, are taken into account.

In England and Wales if there is no legal proxy, close relative or other person who is willing or able to support or represent the patient and the decision involves serious medical treatment, the doctor must approach their employing or contracting organisation about appointing an Independent Mental Capacity Advocate (IMCA), as required by the Mental Capacity Act 2005. The IMCA has the authority to make enquiries about the patient and contribute to the decision by representing the patient's interests, but cannot make a decision on behalf of the patient. It is good practice to have discussions with patients regarding treatment and care towards the end of life to ensure timely access to safe, effective care and continuity in its delivery to meet the patient's needs. An advance care plan can be formulated in which patients document their wishes regarding treatment. This can encompass advance refusals of treatment (which are legally binding) and requests for certain treatments, but the overall decision to administer these treatments lies with the consultant in charge of the patient.

1. The Intensive Care Society Standards Committee. Guidelines for limitations of treatment for adults requiring intensive care. London, UK: ICS, 2003.
2. General Medical Council. Treatment and care towards the end of life: good practice in decision making. London, UK: GMC, 2010.

37 F, F, F, F, T

The Surviving Sepsis Campaign (SSC) guidelines 2012 are an amalgamation of guidelines divided into two care bundles. The first of these is a bundle of resuscitation measures which are recommended to be completed within 3 hours of identification of severe sepsis and include:

* Measurement of lactate level.
* Blood cultures prior to administration of most appropriate antibiotics.
* Administration of broad-spectrum antibiotics.
* Administer 30ml/kg crystalloid for hypotension or lactate ≥4mmol/L.

The second of the sepsis bundles is recommended to be completed within 6 hours and includes the use of vasopressors (for hypotension that does not respond to initial fluid resuscitation) to maintain a mean arterial pressure (MAP) ≥65mmHg or in the event of persistent arterial hypotension despite volume resuscitation (septic shock) or initial lactate ≥4mmol/L.

In the guidelines, the recommended targets for resuscitation are a central venous pressure (CVP) of ≥8mmHg, central venous saturation (ScvO$_2$) of ≥70%, and a normalisation of lactate. The Surviving Sepsis guidelines recommend noradrenaline as the first-line vasopressor in preference to vasopressin.

1.   Surviving Sepsis Campaign: international guidelines for management of severe sepsis and septic shock: 2012. http://www.sccm.org/Documents/SSC-Guidelines.pdf (accessed 24th July 2014).

38   T, F, T, F, F

The CAM-ICU score is a widely validated scoring system for detecting delirium in ICU patients. It assesses the patient for the presence of four features: acute onset or fluctuating course, inattention, altered mental state and disorganised thinking. If the first two features are present plus one of the last two, the patient is 'CAM-ICU positive' and considered to have delirium.

1.   Ely EW, Margolin R, Francis J, et al. Evaluation of delirium in critically ill patients: validation of the Confusion Assessment Method for the Intensive Care Unit (CAM-ICU). Crit Care Med 2001; 29(7): 1370-9.

39   F, T, F, T, F

Functional warm ischaemia time commences when there is inadequate oxygenation or perfusion of the organ as defined by a systolic arterial pressure <50mmHg, oxygen saturation <70% or both, such as during withdrawal of treatment or cardiac standstill and continues until the initiation of cold perfusion. The cold ischaemic time extends from initiation of cold perfusion until restoration of warm circulation after transplantation.

There is no longer an upper or lower age limit to the age of potential donors, although there are organ-specific recommendations for the age of the donor. Kidneys, liver, pancreas, lung and tissue are all suitable for transplantation from donors undergoing donation after cardiac death. Donation after brain death is the only source of hearts for transplantation. Hypotension will occur in most brain-dead donors secondary to relative hypovolaemia exacerbated by reduced systemic vascular resistance. Crystalloid or colloid infusions should be titrated to achieve euvolaemia. Early restoration of vascular tone aids haemodynamic stability and helps reduce the risk of excessive fluid administration.

Vasopressin is considered as the first-line agent where hypotension is resistant to fluid therapy. It restores vascular tone, treats diabetes insipidus, minimises catecholamine requirements, and is less likely than noradrenaline to cause metabolic acidosis or pulmonary hypertension. In some centres, dopamine is the preferred agent and it is important to be aware of local policy when instituting such therapies.

1.   Dunne K, Doherty P. Donation after circulatory death. *Contin Educ Anaesth Crit Care Pain* 2011; 11(3): 82-6.
2.   Gordon JK, McKinlay J. Physiological changes after brain stem death and the management of the heart-beating donor. *Contin Educ Anaesth Crit Care Pain* 2012; 12(5): 225-9.
3.   http://www.bts.org.uk/Documents/Guidelines/Active/DCD%20for%20BTS%20and%20ICS%20FINAL.pdf.

40   T, T, T, F, T

Gram-positive bacteria have an inner cell membrane and an outer thick peptidoglycan layer. This allows the bacteria to take up the purple-coloured Gram stain which is characteristic of Gram-positive species.

Gram-negative bacteria have a thinner peptidoglycan layer surrounded by an outer cell membrane and therefore take up less of the purple stain, retaining the lighter counterstain which is subsequently applied in the Gram-staining process and thus appearing pink on microscopy.

Gram-positive bacteria include *Staphylococci*, *Streptococci*, *Enterococci*, *Corynebacterium*, *Listeria*, *Bacillus* and *Clostridium*.

Gram-negative bacteria include *Haemophilus*, *Neisseria*, *Acinetobacter* and *Enterobacteriaceae*.

1.	Kumar V, Abbas A, Fausto N, Aster J. *Robbins & Cotran Pathologic Basis of Disease*, Professional Edition, 8th ed. Elsevier Publishing, 2009.

41 T, F, T, F, F

In the majority of patients, hyponatraemia is hypotonic such that the effective osmolality and the sodium level are low. In rare cases, the serum contains additional osmoles that render the serum isotonic with osmolality values approaching normal. Causes include hyperglycaemia, mannitol use and glycine absorption during prolonged urological surgery.

Causes of hypotonic hyponatraemia include the syndrome of inappropriate antidiuretic hormone secretion (SIADH), psychogenic polydipsia and cerebral salt wasting syndrome, hypoadrenalism and beer potomania.

1.	Spasovski G, Vanholder R, Allolio B, *et al*. Clinical practice guideline on diagnosis and treatment of hyponatraemia. *Nephrol Dial Transplant* 2014; 29(Suppl 2): i1-39.

42 F, F, T, F, T

The ideal gas laws explain the relationship between a gas's pressure, temperature and volume. Boyle's law states that at a constant temperature, the volume of a given mass of gas varies inversely with pressure. When flying at altitude, atmospheric pressure is less and an ideal gas's volume will increase. Charles' law states that at a constant pressure, the product of temperature and volume is a constant. As the volume of a gas increases with altitude, care must be taken with gas in enclosed body cavities and medical devices. The pressure of the cuff of an endotracheal tube must be monitored or, alternatively, filled with saline. In most modern aircraft with modern navigation systems, defibrillation can be attempted without interference to flight but this must be communicated to the pilots before an attempt is made.

Divers ascending too quickly can develop decompression sickness. As they ascend, nitrogen moves out of solution and bubbles form in joints, skin, muscle and the central nervous system. Flying at altitude will cause more nitrogen to move out of solution and exacerbate this condition. Patients with decompression sickness who require transfer by air should be flown at a maximum flight level of 500ft above mean sea level to keep the effects of altitude to a minimum.

Acceleration forces experienced in routine helicopter operations tend to be of low magnitude and are little different from those experienced in road transfers. In fixed-wing vehicles, acceleration and deceleration forces can be significant on take-off and landing.

1.   Johnson D, Luscombe M. Aeromedical transfer of the critically ill patient. *J Intensive Care Soc* 2011; 12(4): 307-12.

43   F, T, F, T, T

Hypothermia is defined as a core body temperature of less than 35°C. Mild hypothermia is 32-35°C. Moderate hypothermia is 29-32°C and severe hypothermia is less than 29°C.

Hypothermia may produce the following ECG changes:

* Bradyarrhythmias such as sinus bradycardia, AV block, atrial fibrillation with slow ventricular response and slow junctional rhythms.
* Osborn (J) waves.
* Artifact due to shivering.
* Prolonged PR, QRS and QT intervals.
* Ventricular ectopics.
* Cardiac arrest due to asystole, ventricular fibrillation (VF) or ventricular tachycardia (VT).

The Osborn or J-wave is a convex positive deflection (negative deflection in avR and V1) at the junction of the QRS complex and the ST segment (known as the J-point). It is usually more prominent in the precordial leads. It is suggestive of hypothermia and appears at temperatures below 33°C. However, the J-waves are not pathognomonic for hypothermia and can occur in hypercalcaemia and intracranial hypertension, head injuries and subarachnoid haemorrhage. The J-wave may be a normal variant.

1.   Wagner, GS. *Marriott's Practical Electrocardiography*, 11th ed. Lippincott Williams & Wilkins, 2007.
2.   Hampton JR. *The ECG in Practice*, 5th ed. Churchill Livingstone, 2008.

44   T, F, F, F, F

Severe hyponatraemia is dependent on symptoms, characterised by either seizures, decreased conscious level, cardiorespiratory distress or vomiting. Profound hyponatraemia refers to biochemical severity and denotes a serum sodium <125mmol/L.

Recent guidance produced by the European Society for Intensive Care Medicine and the European Society for Endocrinology has suggested a slightly more aggressive approach than previous to the management of symptomatic or profound hyponatraemia. Hypertonic 3% saline is advocated by 150ml aliquot regardless of chronicity with the aim to increase serum sodium by 5mmol/L in an attempt to improve symptoms and limit further brain injury. There are clear recommendations against the use of demeclocycline and vasopressin receptor antagonists such as conivaptan.

Desmopressin is a synthetic ADH utilised in the management of diabetes insipidus to promote water retention and would thus exacerbate hypotonic hyponatraemia. Fludrocortisone plays no role in the management of this condition.

1. Spasovski G, Vanholder R, Allolio B, *et al.* Clinical practice guideline on diagnosis and treatment of hyponatraemia. *Nephrol Dial Transplant* 2014; 29(Suppl 2): i1-39.

45   T, F, F, T, T

As part of infection control the World Health Organization has produced guidance called "Your 5 Moments for Hand Hygiene". The five moments are before touching the patient, before clean/aseptic procedure, after body fluid exposure risk, after touching the patient and after touching the patient's surroundings.

Matching Michigan was a quality improvement project based on a model developed in the United States which, over 18 months, saved around 1500 patient lives. It involved the introduction of interventions, which when applied together significantly reduced the incidence of central venous catheter bloodstream infections. In the United Kingdom its implementation was led by the National Patient Safety Agency.

Sterilisation destroys all micro-organisms, including bacterial spores and is achieved using steam, pressure, dry heat or certain chemical sterilants, (glutaraldehyde, phenol and hydrogen peroxide). High-level disinfection destroys all micro-organisms except high numbers of bacterial spores. This is achieved by pasteurisation or using high-level disinfectants, e.g. chlorhexidine, glutaraldehyde and hydrogen peroxide (at a lesser concentration than that required to perform sterilisation). Intermediate and low-level disinfection involves liquid contact with hospital disinfectants which destroys vegetative bacteria, mycobacteria, most viruses, and most fungi, but not bacterial spores. 2% chlorhexidine in 70% isopropyl alcohol should be used for skin preparation prior to central venous catheter insertion; however, it disinfects the skin rather than sterilising it.

Critical items are those associated with a high risk of infection which contact sterile tissue. These must be sterilised, either by steam or liquid chemical methods. Semi-critical items (including laryngoscope blades, endoscopes, bronchoscopes) come into contact with mucous membranes or non-intact skin and should be disinfected using liquid chemical methods before use. Non-critical items (including blood pressure cuffs, saturation probes, bed rails, bedside tables) come into contact with intact skin but not mucous membranes. They are decontaminated using low-level disinfectants.

1.   World Health Organization. Your 5 Moments for Hand Hygiene. WHO 2009. http://www.who.int/gpsc/5may/Your_5_Moments_For_Hand_Hygiene_Poster.pdf (accessed 21st July 2014).

2.   The Matching Michigan Collaboration & Writing Committee. 'Matching Michigan': a 2-year stepped interventional programme to minimise central venous catheter-blood stream infections in intensive care units in England. *Br Med J Qual Saf* 2013; 22(2): 110-23.

3.   Rutala WA, Weber DJ. Disinfection and sterilization in health care facilities: what clinicians need to know. *Clin Infect Dis* 2004; 39: 702-9.

4.   Loveday HP, Wilson JA, Pratt RJ, *et al.* epic3: national evidence-based guidelines for preventing healthcare-associated infections in NHS hospitals in England. *J Hosp Infect* 2014; 86S1: S1-70.

46   T, F, T, F, T

Approximately 12-20% of individuals presenting with an aortic dissection have a 'normal' chest X-ray; therefore, a normal film does NOT rule out aortic dissection.

Very often widening of the mediastinum is often thought of as being due to aortic dissection. This radiological sign has moderate sensitivity in the setting of an ascending aortic dissection. However, it has low specificity, as many other conditions can cause a widening of the mediastinum on chest X-ray, such as a mediastinal mass, oesophageal rupture, aortic folding and pericardial effusion.

Pleural effusions may also be seen on chest X-ray. They are more commonly seen in descending aortic dissections. If seen, they are typically left-sided pleural effusions.

Other findings include obliteration of the aortic knob, depression of the left mainstem bronchus, loss of the paratracheal stripe, and tracheal deviation.

The calcium sign is a finding on chest X-ray that suggests aortic dissection. It is the separation of the intimal calcification from the outer aortic soft tissue border by 10mm.

1.   Kamalakannan D, Rosman HS, Eagle KA. Acute aortic dissection. *Crit Care Clin* 2007; 23(4): 779-800.

47   F, F, F, T, F

Necrotising fasciitis is a life-threatening soft tissue infection that requires early detection and prompt aggressive multimodal treatment to maximise chances of survival.

The disease is most commonly classified by a microbial source of infection with Type 1 as polymicrobial being the most common, Type 2 monomicrobial, Type 3 Gram-negative marine-related organisms and Type 4 fungal.

Antimicrobial therapy is bactericidal but is also focused on the termination of toxin production and systemic effect. Usually an agent such as clindamycin or linezolid performs this latter role in addition to a broad-spectrum agent such as piperacillin/tazobactam or meropenem.

The Laboratory Risk Indicator for Necrotising Fasciitis Score is designed to distinguish necrotising fasciitis from other soft tissue infections. The score incorporates assessment of C-reactive protein, white cell count, haemoglobin, sodium, creatinine and glucose. A score of > or equal to 8 has a positive predictive value of >90%.

The role of hyperbaric oxygen is controversial. Evidence in support is limited and multiple logistic concerns exist with transfer to hyperbaric chambers. As such it cannot be routinely recommended at the present time and should be considered on a case by case basis.

1.   Davoudian P, Flint NJ. Necrotising fasciitis. *Contin Educ Anaesth Crit Care Pain* 2012; 12(5): 245-50.
2.   Wong CH, Khin LW, Heng KS. The LRINEC (Laboratory Risk Indicator for Necrotizing Fasciitis) score: a tool for distinguishing necrotizing fasciitis from other soft tissue infections. *Crit Care Med* 2004; 32: 1535-41.

48   T, T, T, T, T

Infectious diseases and contamination with chemicals or radiation can threaten health of the individual and that of the population as a whole. Notification enables the prompt investigation, risk assessment and response to cases of infectious disease and contamination that present, or could present, a significant risk to human health. As a duty of care, medical practitioners must notify the proper officer of the local authority of patients in whom they have 'reasonable grounds for suspecting' or a firm diagnosis of infectious diseases which have been deemed to be a serious threat to the health of the population. Both bacterial and viral meningitis are notifiable. Acute infectious hepatitis is notifiable; this includes hepatitis A, B and C. Close contacts of acute hepatitis A and B cases need rapid prophylaxis and urgent notification will facilitate prompt laboratory testing. Hepatitis C cases known to be acute need to be followed up rapidly as this may signify recent transmission from a source that could be controlled.

1.   Department of Health. 13698. Health protection legislation guidance 2010. London, UK: DoH, 2010.

49   T, F, F, F, T

Acute compartment syndrome is a limb-threatening problem. It results from pressure increases within a fascia-bound muscular compartment, with consequent compression of the structures within the compartment including nerves and blood vessels. It can affect many parts of the body; the forearm (volar compartment) and leg (anterior compartment) are most commonly affected. Compartment syndrome of the deep posterior (leg) compartment of the leg is easily missed as this part of the body may not be easily examined. Limb pain is often increased by passive stretching.

Limb compartment syndrome is most commonly caused by fractures (in approximately 75% of cases) with a highest incidence in tibial fractures. Other causes include: burns; seizures; crush injuries; prolonged or excessive exertion; long periods of immobilisation and extravasation of intravenous substances. Due to the risk of bleeding into compartments, patients with a coagulopathy are at particular risk of compartment syndrome.

A limb affected by compartment syndrome may still have palpable distal pulses and normal capillary refill, and it should be noted that complete loss of pulses is often a late sign and should not be relied upon for diagnosis. The use of pulse oximetry is insensitive and is of limited use as a diagnostic tool. Tissue pressure should be measured in the compartments of the at-risk limb. The normal tissue pressures range between 0 and 10mmHg. Capillary blood flow within the compartment can be compromised at pressures >20mmHg. At pressures >30-40mmHg the risk of necrosis is increased. The compartment pressure measurement should be used to guide the need for a fasciotomy to relieve the compartment pressures by allowing expansion of the contents within.

1. Newton EJ, Love J. Acute complications of extremity trauma. *Emerg Med Clin North Am* 2007; 25(3): 751-61.
2. Farrow C, Bodenham A, Troxler M. Acute limb compartment syndromes. *Contin Educ Anaesth Crit Care Pain* 2011; 11(1): 24-8.

50   T, F, T, T, F

Serum and urinary neutrophil gelatinase-associated lipoprotein (NGAL), along with serum cystatin C and urinary Kim-1, have all been recently highlighted as having the potential to identify acute kidney injury (AKI) earlier than standard biomarkers, and with higher sensitivity. N-acetyl cysteine has been the subject of much attention regarding use as a nephroprotective agent, but no good evidence exists to support benefit following the onset of AKI.

The Kidney Disease: Improving Global Outcomes (KDIGO) and Risk, Injury, Failure, Loss, End-stage renal disease (RIFLE) criteria to stage the severity of acute kidney disease share many features, including the proportional rise of serum creatinine from baseline and degree of oliguria. There is a very real risk of progression to chronic kidney disease (CKD) in critically ill patients with AKI, as seen in several large studies.

Starch solutions have been the subject of much attention recently and retracted from clinical use in the UK following a Medicines and Healthcare Products Regulatory Agency (MHRA) recommendation. Several randomised trials and a recent systematic review have suggested an increased incidence of renal replacement therapy with use.

1.   Bellomo R, Kellum JA, Ronco C. Acute kidney injury. *Lancet* 2012; 380(9843): 756-66.
2.   http://www.kdigo.org/clinical_practice_guidelines/pdf/KDIGO%20AKI% 20Guideline.pdf (accessed 30th June 2014).
3.   Coca SG, Yusuf B, Shlipak MG, *et al*. Long-term risk of mortality and other adverse outcomes after acute kidney injury: a systematic review and meta-analysis. *Am J Kidney Dis* 2009; 53: 961-73.
4.   Dart AB, Mutter TC, Ruth CA, Taback SP. Hydroxyethyl starch versus other fluid therapies: effects on kidney function. *Cochrane Database Syst Rev* 2013; 7: CD007594.

51   T, F, F, F, F

Ohm's law relates voltage, current and resistance such that:

V (potential difference - Volts) = I (current - Ampere) x R (resistance - Ohms)

The pathophysiological effects of current flowing through the body depend on the voltage and the electrical resistance of the body, most of which occurs in the skin. Dry skin has a resistance in excess of 100,000 Ohms; however, wet skin has a resistance of just 100 Ohms. The extent of injury also depends on the duration of the current, the type of current and the tissues traversed by the current. Currents >10mA cause tetany (cannot let go) and >100mA cause macroshock and can cause ventricular fibrillation. The risk of ventricular fibrillation is greatest if the current passes through the myocardium during the repolarisation of the myocardium, corresponding to the early part of the T-wave on the ECG. If the electric current passes directly through the heart itself, a much smaller current can produce the same current density as a larger current passing through the body and hence ventricular fibrillation may be induced, termed 'microshock'. Equipment used with electrodes, which may contact the heart directly, is termed Type CF, indicating that it is for cardiac use and has a floating circuit. The leakage through its intracardiac connection must be under 50μA, even if it is operating with a single fault. Other medical monitoring equipment is termed Type B, or Type BF, if it has a floating circuit. The maximum permitted patient leakage current is 500μA under single fault conditions.

1.   Bersten AD, Soni N. *Oh's Intensive Care Manual*, 6th ed. Philadelphia, USA: Butterworth Heinemann, Elsevier, 2009.
2.   Davis PD, Kenny GNC, Eds. *Basic Physics and Measurement in Anaesthesia,* 5th ed. USA: Butterworth-Heinemann, 2003.

52   F, T, F, F, T

The accepted diagnostic criteria for diabetic ketoacidosis are:

* Blood glucose >11mmol/L or known diabetes mellitus.
* Ketonaemia >3.0mmol/L or significant ketonuria.
* Plasma bicarbonate <15mmol/L and/or venous pH <7.3.

While the osmolarity is often mildly raised in DKA, a very high value is more in keeping with hyperosmolar hyperglycaemic state (HHS).

1.   Joint British Diabetes Societies Inpatient Care Group. The management of diabetic ketoacidosis in adults, 2nd ed. London, UK: Joint British Diabetes Societies Inpatient Care Group for NHS Diabetes, 2013.

53   F, T, F, F, T

Amylase >3 times the upper limit of normal is a diagnostic criterion. The Atlanta classification also goes on to define acuity and severity, using the definition of transient organ failure (defined as <48h) to guide prognostication.

The Marshall severity scoring system is a clinical assessment tool and contains renal, cardiovascular and respiratory indices. Balthazar grading refers to radiological assessment of severity and identification of necrosis. The British Society of Gastroenterology has previously identified lipase as a superior test and has recommended its use over serum amylase since 2005.

1.	Banks PA, Bollen TL, Dervenis C, et al. Classification of acute pancreatitis - 2012: revision of the Atlanta classification and definitions by international consensus. Gut 2012; 62(1): 102-11.
2.	UK Working party on acute pancreatitis. UK guidelines for the management of acute pancreatitis. Gut 2005; 54: 1-9.

54   T, F, T, F, F

Direct thrombin inhibitors inhibit fibrin-bound thrombin and free thrombin equally well, thus better suppressing thrombus growth. Thrombin inhibition not only attenuates fibrin formation but also reduces thrombin generation and platelet activation.

Dabigatran is an oral direct thrombin inhibitor. It has been shown to be non-inferior to once-daily enoxaparin for thromboprophylaxis after hip or knee arthroplasty and to warfarin for the treatment of venous thromboembolism, and superior to warfarin for the prevention of stroke and systemic embolism in patients with atrial fibrillation. It is administered twice daily and requires no monitoring of effect.

Bivalirudin, lepirudin and hirudin are parenteral direct thrombin inhibitors. The action of bivalirudin is monitored using the activated partial thromboplastin time (aPTT) and its half-life is 25 minutes following intravenous administration.

Danaparoid is a low-molecular-weight heparinoid. It inhibits Factor Xa via antithrombin (it is an indirect Xa inhibitor). It is administered either IV or SC, has a half-life of 24 hours, and is primarily used for the treatment of heparin-induced thrombocytopaenia. Factor X is involved in both the intrinsic and extrinsic pathways of coagulation and when activated (fXa), 1 molecule of fXa can generate >1000 thrombin molecules. Direct fXa inhibitors not only inhibit free fXa but also inhibit fXa assembled within the prothrombinase complex. Fondaparinux binds the antithrombin molecule causing a conformational change, which enhances its activity against fXa, and is therefore an indirect fXa inhibitor. It is given SC and has a half-life of 17 hours, and can therefore be administered once daily. Rivaroxiban is an oral direct fXa inhibitor which has been shown to significantly reduce the incidence of venous thromboembolism post-hip or -knee arthroplasty compared with conventional treatment with enoxaparin.

1.	Eikelboom JW, Weitz JI. New anticoagulants. *Circulation* 2010; 121: 1523-32.

## 55	F, T, F, F, T

Takotsubo cardiomyopathy (TCM) is also known as apical ballooning syndrome or 'broken heart syndrome'. It is characterised by transient systolic dysfunction of the apical and or mid segments of the left ventricle that mimics a myocardial infarction but in the absence of obstructive coronary artery disease. It typically affects women aged over 50 and can be caused by emotional or physically stressful events as well as cocaine use, methamphetamine use or opiate withdrawal. ECG changes can be confused with an ST elevation MI but coronary angiography is normal. Angiography is required for diagnosis as there is no other accurate method to distinguish TCM from acute coronary syndrome using ECG or cardiac markers or echocardiography alone. Treatment includes angiotensin converter enzyme inhibitors (ACE-i), β-blockers and diuretics. It has an excellent prognosis with 95% of patients recovering completely.

1.	Hurst RT, Prasad A, Askew JW, *et al.* Takotsubu cardiomyopathy: a unique cardiomyopathy with variable ventricular morphology. *J Am Coll Cardiol* 2010; 3: 641-9.

## 56	F, T, T, T, F

POSSUM (Physiological and Operative Severity Score for the enUmeration of Mortality and Morbidity) scoring was first published within the literature in 1991 as a retrospective and prospective surgical audit tool, designed to highlight increasing morbidity/mortality and focus clinical effort. It requires input of physiological data and also operative data including operation type, amount of blood loss, presence of malignancy and peritoneal soiling. No postoperative parameters are included and the model can be easily accessed online.

It has since gained momentum with prospective validation and is now used as a risk prediction tool to guide clinical decision making pre-operatively and assist informed consent. If using the tool in this way, however, the clinician is required to estimate intra-operative findings in advance including the degree of blood loss, extent of malignancy and presence of peritoneal contamination. Multiple surgery-specific versions are available, including the V(ascular)-POSSUM and O(oesophagogastric)-POSSUM.

1.   Copeland GP, Jones D, Walters M. POSSUM: a scoring system for surgical audit. *Br J Surg* 1991; 78(3): 355-60.
2.   Merad F, Baron G, Pasquet B, *et al*. Prospective evaluation of in-hospital mortality with the P-POSSUM scoring system in patients undergoing major digestive surgery. *World J Surg* 2012; 36(10): 2320-7.

57   F, F, T, F, F

When air enters the trachea at the larynx it is already warmed to 34°C with a relative humidity of 88%. By the time it reaches the carina it is 35°C and has 91% relative humidity. It is not until it reaches the first division of the bronchi that it reaches 37°C and 100% relative humidity. The principal function of heat and moisture exchangers (HMEs) is to capture moisture from expired respiratory gases by condensation on the material of the element, and to return this to dry inspired gases providing humidification. HMEs can achieve a relative humidity of 60-70% with gas temperatures of 28°C. Hot-water humidifiers either pass gas over (i.e. blow-by humidifier) or through (i.e. bubble or cascade humidifier) a heated water reservoir. The temperature of the bath is thermostatically controlled and a heated wire may be sited in the inspiratory tubing to achieve the delivery of a gas with a relative humidity of 100% at 37°C. Sidestream nebulisers use an extrinsic gas flow and the Bernoulli principle to draw the drug mixture into the inspiratory flow. The additional gas flow may impair ventilator triggering since it may prevent the development of a negative pressure or cause a reduction in the continuous flow needed to trigger ventilation. Ultrasonic nebulisers, however, do not alter the tidal volume or have an effect on ventilator triggering. Nebuliser deposition is variable. Studies have shown that delivery of the charge ranged from 6-37%, depending upon humidification and breath activation. Placement of the nebuliser on the inspiratory limb, breath activation, use of a large chamber, tidal volumes of 500ml or more and minimisation of turbulent inspiratory flow augment aerosol delivery.

1. Hutton P, Cooper GM, James III FM, Butterworth IV JF. *Fundamental Principles and Practice of Anaesthesia*. London, UK: Martin Dunitz, 2002.
2. Bersten AD, Soni N. *Oh's Intensive Care Manual*, 6th ed. Philadelphia, USA: Butterworth Heinemann, Elsevier, 2009.

58   T, T, F, F, F

Carbon monoxide poisoning can lead to insufficient muscle energy production causing rhabdomyolysis. As muscles are broken down, myoglobin is released. These can form casts and cause obstruction at the glomeruli. This can be reduced by alkalinisation of urine to keep the pH above 7. Calcium levels can drop in the acute phase but later can be sequestered in muscles so low levels should ideally not be replaced unless the patient is symptomatic. Although mannitol is sometimes advocated to promote diuresis and flush out precipitated myoglobin from the kidneys, there is no high quality evidence that it reduces the incidence of renal failure due to rhabdomyolysis.

1. Lerma EV, Berns JS, Nissenson SR. *Current Diagnosis and Treatment, Nephrology and Hypertension*. McGraw-Hill Companies, 2009: 109-12.

59   T, F, T, F, F

Although the pH is fairly normal, there is significant physiological disturbance. This patient has a significant hypoalbuminaemic alkalosis, hyperchloraemic acidosis and hypernatraemic (contraction) alkalosis despite an apparently minimally deranged blood gas. The chloride is high causing a degree of metabolic acidosis (reducing the strong ion difference [SID]), offset slightly by the high Na (overall effect equivalent to a base deficit of -5). The base deficit needs to be adjusted for the low albumin (correction: 0.25meq/L per drop of 4g/L albumin below 42); an albumin of 6 corresponds to a base deficit of ([42-6]/4) x 0.25 = -9. SID is Na+K+Ca+Mg-Cl and a normal value is 40-44mEq/L.

1.   Neligan P. Acid-base balance in critical care medicine. http://www.ccmtutorials.com/ renal/Acid%20Base%20Balance%20in%20Critical%20Care%20Medicine-NELIGAN.pdf (accessed 29th September 2014).

60 F, T, T, F, F

Hypertension is one of the most important preventable causes of premature morbidity and mortality in the UK and is a major risk factor for ischaemic and haemorrhagic stroke, myocardial infarction, heart failure, chronic kidney disease, cognitive decline and death. The Joint National Committee (JNC) on Prevention, Detection, Evaluation, and Treatment of High Blood Pressure categorises blood pressure as outlined in Table 2.2.

Table 2.2. JNC classification of arterial blood pressure in adults.

BP Class	Systolic BP (mmHg)	Diastolic BP (mmHg)
Normal	<120	<80
Prehypertension	121-139	80-89
Stage I	140-159	90-99
Stage II	>159	>99
Hypertensive crisis	>179	>109

Hypertension is diagnosed from an average of two or more readings taken more than 1 minute apart or using 24 monitoring or home measurements. The two readings can take place at the same visit to the doctor and if severe hypertension is diagnosed, antihypertensives should be considered without waiting for confirmatory ambulatory monitoring. Antihypertensive treatment consists of a step-wise increase in doses and numbers of medications. When optimal or maximum tolerated doses of an ACE inhibitor or angiotensin receptor antagonist, calcium channel blocker and a diuretic are given and the patient remains hypertensive with a BP >140/90mmHg, resistant hypertension is diagnosed. A fourth antihypertensive and/or seeking expert advice should be considered. Severe elevation in BP with evidence of end-organ damage is classified as a 'hypertensive emergency'; when no end-organ damage is seen, 'hypertensive urgency' is diagnosed. Patients with a hypertensive emergency should have their BP lowered immediately, although not to 'normal' levels, whereas patients with urgency should have their BP lowered over 24-48 hours to avoid disrupting brain blood flow autoregulation.

1. National Institute for Health and Care Excellence. Hypertension. NICE clinical guideline 127. London, UK: NICE, 2013. www.nice.org.uk (accessed 25th February 2015).
2. Marik PE, Varon J. Hypertensive crises: challenges and management. *Chest* 2007; 131(6): 1949-62.
3. The Seventh Report of the Joint National Committee on Prevention, Detection, Evaluation, and Treatment of High Blood Pressure. http://www.nhlbi.nih.gov/files/docs/guidelines/jnc7full.pdf (accessed 2nd January 2015).

61 A

Numerous routes of drug delivery are possible, but in this situation the best will be the one that can be achieved rapidly while ensuring reliable delivery of arrest drugs. The latest International Liaison Committee on Resuscitation (ILCOR) guidelines recommend intraosseous access which is usually quick to obtain and guarantees access of drugs to the circulation. Intramuscular absorption of drugs will be poor given the poor peripheral circulation in cardiac arrest even with good cardiopulmonary resuscitation; surgical cutdown and central venous catheter insertion will both provide guaranteed access to the circulation but will take time to achieve and require an experienced operator. Drug administration down the endotracheal tube is no longer recommended due to uncertainty about dose and reliability of absorption into the circulation.

1.   Resuscitation Council (UK). Advanced life support 2011. London, UK: Resuscitation Council (UK). https://www.resus.org.uk/pages/als.pdf (accessed 25th February 2015).

62   D

Extracorporeal membrane oxygenation has increasingly gained favour for the management of refractory respiratory failure, following the results of the CESAR (Conventional ventilation or ECMO for Severe Adult Respiratory failure) trial and the increased use during the 2009 swine flu pandemic. Several positively slanted review articles assessing critical care utilisation are available. However, it is an intervention not without cost and risk implications. As such, it must be considered carefully and the evidence appraised objectively.

In the assessor-blinded prospective multicentre CESAR trial, 90 patients of 180 were randomised to receive ECMO compared to conventional support at the referring hospital. However, only three quarters of these patients actually received the intervention (68/90). As such, the mortality difference reported (relative risk 0·69; 95% CI 0·05-0·97; p=0·03) reflects the transfer of patients to a specialist respiratory centre with the capacity for ECMO, rather than a direct effect of the intervention itself.

ECMO can be administered via arteriovenous supply (with propulsion cardiovascular support) or venovenous for assistance with gas exchange only. Respiratory ECMO has been noted in cohort studies to result in survival rates of >50% on average, with graft failure listed as a common indication. Extracorporeal cardiopulmonary resuscitation is indeed gaining favour for refractory cardiac arrest in the young, with some developing anecdotal literature. Vascular access issues and terminal diagnoses require careful consideration of both risk and cost prior to use. Patients with cardiogenic shock will gain little benefit from venovenous ECMO but may benefit from veno-arterial ECMO if the cardiac function is potentially reversible.

1. Hung M, Vuylsteke A, Valchanov K. Extracorporeal membrane oxygenation: coming to an ICU near you. *J Intensive Care Soc* 2012; 13(1): 31-8.
2. Peek GJ, Mugford M, Tiruvoipati R, *et al*. Efficacy and economic assessment of conventional ventilatory support versus extracorporeal membrane oxygenation for severe adult respiratory failure (CESAR): a multicentre randomised controlled trial. *Lancet* 2009; 374(9698): 1351-63.
3. Chen YS, Lin JW, Yu HY, *et al*. Cardiopulmonary resuscitation with assisted extracorporeal life-support versus conventional cardiopulmonary resuscitation in adults with in-hospital cardiac arrest: an observational study and propensity analysis. *Lancet* 2008; 372 (9638): 554-61.

63 E

Magnesium is the second most abundant intracellular cation and the fourth most abundant cation in the body. It is an important co-factor for many biological processes and is an essential mineral that is important for bone mineralisation, muscular relaxation, neurotransmission, and other cell functions. Causes of hypomagnesaemia include excess loss (polyuria of any cause, severe diarrhoea, prolonged vomiting and large nasogastric aspirates) and inadequate intake (starvation, parenteral nutrition, alcoholism and malabsorption syndromes). Clinical features include confusion, irritability, seizures, weakness and lethargy, arrhythmias and symptoms related to hypocalcaemia and hypokalaemia which are resistant to calcium and potassium supplementation, respectively. The combination of symptomatic signs of hypocalcaemia, hypokalaemia and hypomagnesaemia mean intravenous magnesium replacement should be the first-line therapy.

1. Martin KJ, Gonzalez EA, Slatopolsky E. Clinical consequences and management of hypomagnesemia. *J Am Soc Nephrol* 2009; 20: 2291-5.
2. Singer M, Webb AR, Eds. *Oxford Handbook of Critical Care*, 2nd ed. USA: Oxford University Press, 2005.

64 C

Listeria monocytogenes is an important causative organism for disease in the elderly, immunocompromised or pregnant patient, and a high index of suspicion is required in these groups. It may also cause problems in otherwise healthy individuals. Diarrhoea is a common symptom but meningitis is a more serious clinical presentation. Patients may present with focal seizures and the disease may have a more insidious onset compared with other forms of bacterial meningitis. Blood cultures are positive in 60-75% of patients with CNS *Listeria* infections. *Listeria* organisms show a characteristic flagellar-driven 'tumbling' motility pattern in wet mounts of cerebrospinal fluid (CSF). CSF analysis shows a pleocytosis, with moderately high protein levels. In *Cryptococcus* infection, the CSF protein levels would be very high so this goes against the diagnosis here. CSF glucose levels in *Listeria* infection can be low and this is associated with a poor prognosis. In the question, the low glucose goes against viral meningitis. Ampicillin is used as part of *Listeria* treatment; gentamicin is often added for synergy, but may be stopped after clinical improvement in order to decrease the chance of nephrotoxicity or ototoxicity.

1.	Weinstein KB. *Listeria monocytogenes*. http://www.emedicine.medscape.com/article/220684-overview (accessed 29th July 2014).

65   C

Use of the prone position for refractory hypoxaemia in acute respiratory distress syndrome (ARDS) has gained favour in recent years. Previous data demonstrated physiological improvement via surrogate endpoints, but limited impact on hard outcomes. In 2013, the well-conducted PROSEVA (Proning Severe ARDS patients) trial managed to demonstrate a statistically significant reduction in death at both 28 and 90 days with 16-hour sessions in the prone position for patients with severe ARDS. As such, use of the prone position is rapidly becoming a standard of care for those patients with a P/F ratio of <20kPa (<150mmHg). Intensivists should be well aware of the complications and risk/benefit analysis.

A supplementary appendix for the PROSEVA trial provides data on many complications. Interestingly, there was no difference in the rate of mainstem bronchus intubations, although the rate of endotracheal tube obstruction doubled in the prone group. There was no difference in the rates of cardiac arrest between groups.

A further paper has gone on to analyse the rate of pressure sores in patients turned prone, which are significantly increased when compared to those nursed in the supine position. This risk is likely to be outweighed by the significant mortality benefit and as such should be an expected complication, although vigilance and reflection to continually minimise harm should be frequent.

None of the other interventions listed has been shown to improve mortality in randomised controlled trials.

1. Curley MA. Prone positioning of patients with acute respiratory distress syndrome: a systematic review. *Am J Crit Care* 1999; 8(6): 397-405.
2. Guérin C, Reignier J, Richard JC, *et al*. Prone positioning in severe acute respiratory distress syndrome. *N Engl J Med* 2013; 368: 2159-68.
3. Girard R, Baboi L, Ayzac L, *et al*. The impact of patient positioning on pressure ulcers in patients with severe ARDS: results from a multicenter randomized controlled trial on prone positioning. *Intensive Care Med* 2014; 40(3): 397-403.

66 B

This man has severe sepsis and has evidence of sepsis-induced tissue hypoperfusion. He has been resuscitated with approximately 30ml/kg crystalloid solution and his haemodynamic parameters have improved. As long as there is improvement in the haemodynamic variables, a further fluid challenge should be administered, targeting a MAP of 65mmHg. This fluid challenge may be given as crystalloid or albumin; starches should be avoided. Should he remain hypotensive and become unresponsive to fluids, noradrenaline should be started.

Following fluid optimisation, if plasma lactate remains elevated (signifying ongoing tissue hypoperfusion), the current Surviving Sepsis Campaign guidelines advocate transfusing blood to achieve a haemoglobin concentration of 90g/L to improve oxygen delivery. Of note, a recent large multicentre trial has found no benefit between targeting a haemoglobin of

70g/L and 90g/L in patients with septic shock, so this guidance may change in due course.

Once tissue hypoperfusion has resolved and in the absence of extenuating circumstances (such as myocardial ischaemia, severe hypoxaemia, acute haemorrhage, or ischaemic coronary artery disease), red blood cell transfusion should occur when the haemoglobin concentration decreases to less than 70g/L to target a haemoglobin concentration of 70-90g/L. Blood cultures should be taken and antibiotics administered within the first hour of resuscitation but efforts to stabilise the patient must take precedence. Source control of the infection should take place within the first 12 hours after the diagnosis has been made.

1.	Dellinger RP, Levy MM, Rhodes A, *et al*. Surviving Sepsis Campaign: international guidelines for management of severe sepsis and septic shock: 2012. *Crit Care Med* 2013; 41(2): 580-637.
2.	Holst LB, Haase N, Wetterslev J, *et al*. Lower versus higher haemoglobin threshold for transfusion in septic shock. *New Engl J Med* 2014; 371: 1381-91.

## 67	A

Right ventricular (RV) infarction should always be considered in any patient who has inferior wall myocardial infarction and associated hypotension, especially in the absence of crepitations. There are usually elevated right atrial pressures secondary to the RV infarct. Such patients depend on adequate pre-load and administering intravenous diuretics or nitrates may reduce this with adverse consequences. Slow intravenous fluids may be needed as a temporary measure but the most important step is discussion with the local cardiac centre to discuss possible coronary reperfusion, as he has ongoing chest pain. If too unstable to transfer, urgent thrombolysis may be needed.

1.	Dima C. Right ventricular infarction. http://www.emedicine.medscape.com/article/157961 (accessed 2nd August 2014).

68   A

An understanding of the accuracy, reliability and pragmatic utility of scoring systems is essential to critical care practice. Originally released for use in 1985, the APACHE II score remains widely utilised as a severity scoring system to categorise acuity of patients admitted and influence interpretation of adjusted mortality data. It is a good example from which to develop understanding.

The 12 key variables include temperature, age, MAP, pulse, respiratory rate, sodium, potassium, creatinine, haematocrit, white cell count, GCS and oxygenation. In addition, weight is given to the presence or absence of prescriptive definitions of chronic organ failure and immunocompromise, alongside the need for emergency or elective surgery. Variables are weighted from 1 to 4 with a maximum overall score of 71. The score is calculated based on the worst variables within the first 24 hours of admission. A score of >25 represents a predicted mortality of 50%. Other scoring systems are available.

Validity represents the ability of the score to accurately predict what you want it to predict – in this case mortality. This can also be referred to as calibration. Hence, the APACHE II score is only of use if a higher score correlates with a higher mortality. If the scoring system does not perform well in this regard, it is essentially useless despite other redeeming characteristics.

Generalisability refers to the ability to replicate similar results with the scoring systems across international cohorts. Easy formulae are best, but many use complex statistical models. This is no major issue, provided simple online calculators are provided which allow you to enter basic data only. Discrimination refers to the accuracy of the test, usually defined as an assessment of sensitivity and specificity at multiple cut-off levels followed by a receiving operator characteristic (ROC) curve. The area under this curve defines the test performance ranging from weak to excellent. Although this is important, if the test is not valid, then it is only accurate at predicting something of little interest.

Simple variables are important, but if the test has good validity and discrimination, the addition of complex variables can often provide very useful information.

1. Knaus WA, Draper EA, Wagner DP, Zimmerman JE. APACHE II: a severity of disease classification system *Crit Care Med* 1985; 13(10): 818-29.
2. Bouch DC, Thompson JP. Severity scoring systems in the critically ill. *Contin Educ Anaesth Crit Care Pain* 2008; 8(5): 181-5.

69 A

Ethylene glycol is a clear, odourless liquid with a sweet taste. It is used commercially as antifreeze and de-icer. When ingested it is rapidly absorbed and toxic metabolites cause ocular toxicity, metabolic acidosis and renal failure. Features of intoxication include dizziness, drowsiness, nausea and vomiting, and abdominal pain through to metabolic acidosis, coma and convulsions. Intoxication with ethylene glycol produces a high anion gap metabolic acidosis with hyperosmolality. Specific treatment of ethylene glycol intoxication involves the administration of fomepizole, and if this is not available, ethanol to prevent the further metabolism of ethylene glycol to toxic metabolites. Bicarbonate administration and renal replacement therapy may be required.

Metabolic acidosis is a feature of salicylate intoxication but the osmolal gap would not be raised. Severe tricyclic antidepressant overdose would also cause a metabolic acidosis; however, the QRS duration would likely be prolonged. Cyanide toxicity is rapidly fatal and features include coma, respiratory depression, hypotension and metabolic acidosis. Again hyperosmolality is not a feature. Paraquat causes gastrointestinal pain and vomiting. Dyspnoea and pulmonary oedema occur within 24 hours progressing to irreversible fibrosis and death.

Normal serum osmolarity is 285-290mOsm/L. Serum osmolarity can be calculated using the following equation:

Serum osmolarity (mOsm/L) = 2 x Na^+ (mmol/L) + blood urea nitrogen (mmol/L) + serum glucose (mmol/L).

The osmolal gap is the difference between the calculated osmolarity and the measured osmolarity and is usually <10mOsm/L. Accumulation of ethylene glycol in the serum increases the measured serum osmolarity producing an osmolal gap. Other causes of a raised osmolal gap (lactic acidosis, ketoacidosis, renal failure) do not cause an increase in the osmolal gap >20mOsm/L, thus, if this is seen, an alcohol-related intoxication is present.

1. Kraut JA, Kurtz I. Toxic alcohol ingestions: clinical features, diagnosis, and management. *Clin J Am Soc Nephrol* 2008; 3: 208-25.
2. Bersten AD, Soni N. *Oh's Intensive Care Manual*, 6th ed. Philadelphia, USA: Butterworth Heinemann, Elsevier, 2009.

70   A

Acute fatty liver of pregnancy (AFLP) is a relatively rare diagnosis but one associated with a high mortality. Estimated maternal mortality is around 10-20% and a perinatal mortality of 20-30%. These figures are much improved from nearly 20 years ago as early recognition and management have improved. It tends to occur in the third trimester. AFLP is histologically and clinically similar to Reye's syndrome, both diseases of microvesicular fatty infiltration. It is thought to be caused by abnormal oxidation of mitochondrial fatty acids, although the exact pathophysiology remains unclear.

It can coexist with pre-eclampsia. It is characterised by an insidious onset of jaundice, clotting derangement (predominantly raised prothrombin time and decreased fibrinogen level) and a transaminitis (usually not exceeding 1000IU/L). Due to liver glycogen storage being impaired or problems with glycogenolysis, hypoglycaemia is commonly seen and there may be a hepatic encephalopathy seen.

There is not enough in the history to suggest liver haematoma as there would be right upper quadrant pain and more evidence of haemodynamic instability to suggest this and/or a history of trauma.

Cholestasis of pregnancy is commonly seen but the bilirubin would be less than 100µmol/L and is associated with a normal clotting profile.

Viral hepatitis would be associated with much higher levels of transaminase levels and there would be more clues in the history to suggest veno-occlusive disease such as Budd-Chiari syndrome with the classic triad of abdominal pain, ascites and hepatomegaly. This is usually diagnosed by the use of Doppler of the portal vein on ultrasound scanning. Budd-Chiari syndrome tends to occur more frequently in the post-partum state.

1.   World Federation of Societies of Anaesthesiologists. Cowie P, Johnston IG. Acute fatty liver of pregnancy. Anaesthesia Tutorial of the Week 191, August 2010. www.aagbi.org/education/educational-resources/tutorial-week (accessed 26th February 2015).
2.   Gutunpallli SR, Steinberg J. Hepatic disease ad pregnancy: an overview of diagnosis and management. *Crit Care Med* 2005; 33(10): S322-9.

 71 D

This patient has septic shock and has had generous intravenous fluid resuscitation. While he may require further fluid, at this stage he needs vasopressor support.

First choice vasopressor therapy has been explored in the context of several large randomised controlled trials in adults. In SOAP (Sepsis Occurrence in Acutely ill Patients) 2, no difference was noted between the use of dopamine and noradrenaline for the treatment of shock, although a higher rate of adverse events was noted in the dopamine group. In VASST (Vasopressin in Septic Shock Trial), no benefit was seen when adding vasopressin to open label vasopressors compared to additional noradrenaline, although there was no increase in mortality at 90 days when groups were compared. The Surviving Sepsis Campaign guidelines advocate noradrenaline as the vasopressor of choice based in part on the above evidence.

The role of albumin in sepsis resuscitation is controversial. The FEAST (Fluid Expansion As Supportive Therapy) trial has suggested that in a large cohort of African children in resource poor settings, the use of an albumin fluid bolus (as taught on the overwhelming majority of paediatric life support courses) during early resuscitation may increase mortality (relative risk 1.45, 95% CI 1.13-1.86). This should not be extrapolated to the resuscitation of an adult patient in a well-resourced healthcare setting however. There is some evidence that albumin is associated with a better outcome in sepsis resuscitation, and it is weakly recommended by the SSC as a second-line fluid therapy in septic shock.

1. Vincent JL, De Backer D. Circulatory shock. *N Engl J Med* 2013; 369: 1726-34.
2. De Backer D, Biston P, Devriendt J, *et al.* Comparison of dopamine and norepinephrine in the treatment of shock. *N Engl J Med* 2010; 362: 779-89.
3. Russell JA, Walley KR, Singer J, *et al.* Vasopressin versus norepinephrine infusion in patients with septic shock. *N Engl J Med* 2008; 358: 877-87.
4. Maitland K, Kiguli S, Opoka RO, *et al.* Mortality after fluid bolus in African children with severe infection. *N Engl J Med* 2011; 364: 2483-95.
5. Dellinger RP, Levy MM, Rhodes A, *et al.* Surviving Sepsis Campaign: international guidelines for management of severe sepsis and septic shock: 2012. *Crit Care Med* 2013; 41: 580-637.

72   C

Amniotic fluid embolism (AFE) presents with a sudden, profound and unexpected maternal collapse associated with hypotension, hypoxaemia and disseminated intravascular coagulation (DIC), due to amniotic fluid, foetal cells, hair and other debris entering the maternal circulation. Most cases occur during labour, 19% during Caesarean section and 11% following vaginal delivery. Advanced maternal age and multiparity are associated with a higher risk of developing AFE. Presenting symptoms and signs include dyspnoea, cough, headache, chest pain, hypotension, foetal distress, pulmonary oedema, cyanosis, coagulopathy, seizures, uterine atony, bronchospasm and transient hypertension. A full blood count and coagulation demonstrate low haemoglobin and abnormal coagulation. Arterial blood gases may show hypoxaemia. Chest X-ray does not often show any abnormality. ECG may demonstrate a right ventricular strain pattern in the early stages. Diagnostic tests include cytological analysis of central venous blood and broncho-alveolar fluid, sialyl-Tn antigen test, zinc coproporphyrin concentration and serum tryptase concentrations. The key factors in the management of AFE are early recognition, prompt resuscitation and delivery of the foetus.

1. Dedhia JD, Mushambi MC. Amniotic fluid embolism. *Contin Educ Anaesth Crit Care Pain* 2007; 7(5): 152-6.

73 D

The ECG is neither sensitive nor specific enough to diagnose or exclude pulmonary embolism (PE), with up to 18% of patients with PE having a completely normal ECG. Sinus tachycardia, the most common abnormality, is seen in 44% of patients. Complete or incomplete right bundle branch block (RBBB) is associated with increased mortality and is seen in 18% of patients. Right ventricular strain pattern is associated with T-wave inversion in the right precordial leads (V1-4) ± the inferior leads (II, III, aVF). This pattern is seen in up to 34% of patients and is associated with high pulmonary artery pressures. Right axis deviation is seen in 16% of patients. Extreme right axis deviation may occur, with an axis between zero and -90°, giving the appearance of left axis deviation ('pseudo left axis'). The S1Q3T3 pattern is associated with a deep S-wave in lead I, Q-wave in III and an inverted T-wave in III. This classic finding is neither sensitive nor specific for PE and is found in only 20% of patients with PE. Non-specific ST segment and T-wave changes, including ST elevation and depression, are also common.

The causes of these ECG changes may be due to dilation of the right atrium and right ventricle with a resultant shift in the position of the heart, and increased stimulation of the sympathetic nervous system as a result of anxiety, pain and hypoxia, and right ventricular ischaemia.

1.   Kosuge M, Kimura K, Ishikawa T, *et al.* Electrocardiographic differentiation between acute pulmonary embolism and acute coronary syndromes on the bases of negative T waves. *Am J Cardiol* 2007: 99(6): 817-21.

74 B

Myocardial infarction (MI) simply refers to the death of myocardial cells. The causes for this cell death are numerous and not all related to thrombotic pathology. Definitions and subtypes of MI exist to characterise epidemiology, standardise reporting and focus on therapeutic options. To the latter end, it is important for the practising intensivist to be aware of the different causes of MI and their variable management options. Recent consensus guidance and expert definition exists.

Type 1 MI is defined as a spontaneous myocardial infarction, usually a result of ruptured plaque following mural/wall thrombus. This is the presenting acute coronary syndrome requiring antiplatelet therapy and definitive cardiological treatment. An acute intra-operative event of this type would be extremely unfortunate and relatively rare. A Type 2 MI refers to cell death secondary to an ischaemic (supply/demand) imbalance to the myocardium, which can regularly occur in the critically ill patient. Common causes include septic shock, hypoxia and hypovolaemia. Antiplatelet therapy can be counterproductive here and lead to worsening coagulopathy with no direct benefit. A Type 3 infarct represents sudden death attributable to likely spontaneous myocardial ischaemia, in the absence of biomarker corroboration. Types 4 and 5 are associated with percutaneous coronary intervention and coronary artery bypass grafting, respectively.

This patient is most likely to have suffered a Type 2 MI due to intra-operative hypotension and septic shock. Management focuses on optimisation of oxygen delivery via standard means rather than antiplatelet therapy and primary percutaneous coronary intervention.

1.   Thygesen K, Alpert JS, Jaffe AS, *et al*. Third universal definition of acute myocardial infarction. *J Am Coll Cardiol* 2012; 60(16): 1581-98.

75   E

Stress-related mucosal damage is a continuum from superficial erosions to ulcers causing clinically significant bleeding. The prevalence of clinically significant gastrointestinal bleeding amongst the critically ill is reported to be between 0.6-4%. Studies have shown those patients with coagulopathies and those undergoing mechanical ventilation for >48 hours have substantial risk factors for clinically significant bleeding. Sucralfate, histamine-2 receptor blockers and the use of proton pump inhibitors have all been shown to reduce the incidence of stress-related mucosal damage by increasing the pH of gastric secretions. Liquid enteral feed buffers gastric acid, increases mucosal blood flow and induces the secretion of cytoprotective prostaglandins and mucus. Continuous enteral feeding has been shown to be more effective at increasing intragastric pH than histamine-2 receptor blockers and proton pump inhibitors. This patient is maintained on full enteral feed, and as such she does not require additional stress ulcer prophylaxis.

1.   Plummer MP, Blaser AR, Deane AM. Stress ulceration: prevalence, pathology and association with adverse outcomes. *Crit Care* 2014; 18: 213.

76   E

Cocaine stimulates the sympathetic nervous system by inhibiting catecholamine reuptake at sympathetic nerve terminals stimulating central sympathetic outflow and increasing the sensitivity of adrenergic nerve endings to norepinephrine. Cocaine promotes thrombosis by activating platelets and promoting platelet aggregation. Myocardial infarction (MI) in non-cocaine-using patients with traditional risk factors typically results from plaque fissure or rupture with plaque haemorrhage, which precipitates thrombosis. In contrast, MI in cocaine-using patients involves intracoronary thrombosis superimposed on smooth muscle cell-rich fibrous plaques without plaque rupture or haemorrhage. The risk of myocardial infarction rises as much as 24-fold during the first hour after cocaine use. Although the risk decreases significantly after that, cocaine-related vasoconstriction can still cause acute MI hours or as many as 4 days later. If ST elevation MI is suspected in this context, then acute coronary syndrome treatment and discussion with a local primary coronary intervention centre should be considered. Urgent thrombolysis should be considered unless there are any contraindications such as severe hypertension (as in this case), aortic dissection, seizures, etc.

Benzodiazepines may be used first-line, closely followed by nitrate therapy. Calcium channel blockers and phentolamine may also be used. β-blockers are avoided due to unopposed α-agonism. In this case the patient is agitated and hypertensive so a reasonable option would be to sedate the patient with an intravenous benzodiazepine.

1.   McCord J, Jneid H, Hollander JE, *et al*. Management of cocaine-associated chest pain and myocardial infarction. *Circulation* 2008; 117: 1897-907.

2. Schwartz BG, Rezkalla S, Kloner RA, *et al.* Cardiovascular effects of cocaine. *Circulation* 2010; 122: 2558-69.
3. Rezkalla SH, Kloner RA. Cocaine-induced acute myocardial infarction. *Clin Med Res* 2007; 5(3): 172-6.

 77 D

Aortic stenosis is a progressive valvular lesion with additional pathology in the aortic outflow tract and left ventricle, eventually leading to ventricular outflow tract obstruction, cardiovascular collapse and death. It is predominately a disease of the elderly, with a prevalence approaching 10% in patients >80 years of age. Key symptoms include angina, exertional dyspnoea, dizziness, syncope and cardiovascular collapse. Once symptomatic, mortality is approximately 50% at 2 years unless valve replacement is considered promptly.

The disease is progressive and refractory to medical management, although treatment of concurrent disease may improve life expectancy and the chances of successful surgery. Symptoms typically occur when the maximum transvalvular velocity has quadrupled (increased to 4m/second). The disease affects the upstream ventricular outflow tract and the systemic vasculature post-valve, and as such is not truly confined to the leaflets alone. The principles of management include avoiding tachycardia and maintaining a good coronary perfusion pressure, since the left ventricle is hypertrophied and prone to ischaemia should diastolic pressure fall. Drugs which reduce afterload or promote tachycardia should be avoided. A contemporary review article is available.

I. Otto CM, Prendergrast B. Aortic-valve stenosis - from patients at risk to severe valve obstruction. *New Engl J Med* 2014; 371: 744-56.

78 D

Cardiac output monitoring is used in the critically ill patient to guide management in order to optimise tissue oxygenation. Various devices are available to measure or estimate cardiac output, preload variables and central venous saturations. The choice of cardiac output monitor is limited by institutional factors, device-related factors and patient-related factors.

The pulmonary artery catheter (PAC) is the gold standard method of cardiac output monitoring against which all other devices are compared. Cardiac output is measured by intermittent pulmonary artery thermodilution. Pulmonary artery thermodilution cardiac output measurements are unreliable in the presence of tricuspid regurgitation. In general, cardiac output is underestimated in patients with tricuspid regurgitation; therefore, the PAC should be avoided in this case.

Central venous pressure is a poor guide to adequacy of fluid resuscitation even in the absence of tricuspid regurgitation.

Methods of pulse pressure analysis are based on the principle that the stroke volume can be continuously estimated by analysing the arterial pressure waveform. In sinus rhythm, a ventilated patient will have a high stroke volume variation if fluid-responsive, but in a patient with atrial fibrillation the stroke volume variation will be high even if the patient is optimally fluid-loaded.

Bioimpedance uses electric current stimulation for identification of thoracic or body impedance variations induced by cyclic changes in blood flow caused by the heart beating. Evidence to support the use of bioimpedance in haemodynamically unstable patients is yet to be determined.

Oesophageal Doppler use is operator-dependent but studies have shown that only 10-12 insertions are required to obtain accurate measurements. Doppler ultrasound is used to determine the flow of blood through the descending aorta. This is converted into an estimated stroke volume that can be used to assess whether further fluid leads to a significant increase in cardiac output. There are no contraindications in this patient to the use of oesophageal Doppler for cardiac output monitoring and this is the method of choice.

1.   Alhashemi JA, Cecconi M, Hofer CK. Cardiac output monitoring: an integrative perspective. *Crit Care* 2011; 15: 214.

2. Marik PE. Obituary: pulmonary artery catheter 1970 to 2013. *Ann Intens Care* 2013; 3: 38.
3. Drummond KE, Murphy E. Minimally invasive cardiac output monitoring. *Contin Educ Anaesth Crit Care Pain* 2012; 12(1): 5-10.

 79 D

The most likely unifying diagnosis is infectious mononucleosis (glandular fever) due to Ebstein-Barr virus. The organism may cause deranged liver function tests and splenomegaly. The Monospot test is used to diagnose the condition. Sensitivity is 85%, and specificity is 100%. The test may be negative early in the course of EBV infectious mononucleosis. Positivity increases during the first 6 weeks of the illness. This is a heterophile antibody test that relies on the agglutination of horse red blood cells by heterophile antibodies in the patient's serum. The most prominent sign is pharyngitis often with inflamed tonsils and exudate similar to streptococcal infections. Splenomegaly occurs into the second or third week of the condition. Contact sports should be avoided to reduce the risk of splenic rupture.

1. Cunha B. Infectious mononucelosis workup. http://www.emedicine.medscape.com/article/222040-workup (accessed 14th August 2014).
2. Cohen JI. Epstein-Barr infections, including infectious mononucleosis. In: *Harrison's Principles of Internal Medicine*, 17th ed. Kasper DL, Braunwald E, Fauci AS, *et al*. New York, USA: McGraw-Hill Medical Publishing Division, 2008: 380-91.

80 B

Propofol infusion syndrome (PRIS) is a challenging entity, defined as progressive bradydysrhythmias (leading to asystole when untreated) in the presence of either profound metabolic acidosis, hypertriglyceridaemia, rhabdomyolysis or fatty liver. There has been much postulation about the pathophysiology, with current thinking focusing on abnormalities of either mitochondrial fatty acid metabolism or direct respiratory chain inhibition predisposing to intracellular dysfunction and apoptosis. Unexplained metabolic acidosis in the ventilated patient and downsloping ST elevation in the precordial leads are hallmarks of the syndrome, followed by progressive cardiovascular instability. There is a documented association with doses higher than 4mg/kg for >48 hours. In one of the more recent studies looking at >1000 ICU admissions, the incidence of PRIS was recorded as just over 1%. Predisposing factors include young age, catecholamine and glucocorticoid use, critical illness of neurological or respiratory origin and inadequate carbohydrate intake.

1.   Cremer OL. The propofol infusion syndrome: more puzzling evidence on a complex and poorly characterized disorder. *Crit Care* 2009; 13: 1012.

81 D

This patient has moderate *Clostridium difficile* infection and therefore oral metronidazole would be an appropriate agent of choice. However, she has a history of recurrent CDI (3 months ago with recurrence 2 weeks ago and then the current infection), therefore this current infection should be treated with fidaxomicin to decrease the risk of further recurrence.

In addition to the treatment outlined in Table 2.3 below, severe cases of CDI not responding to oral vancomycin, should be treated with high-dose oral vancomycin (up to 500mg qds) +/- IV metronidazole (500mg tds) or oral fidaxomicin (200mg bd). Oral rifampicin or intravenous immunoglobulin can be used but there is no evidence to support the use of these agents. Fidaxomicin is a macrocyclic antibiotic which is given orally and undergoes minimal systemic absorption. It has high faecal concentrations and limited activity against normal gut flora. The side effect profile of fidaxomicin is similar to that of oral vancomycin but it is considerably more expensive. Studies have shown that fidaxomicin is non-inferior to vancomycin in the initial cure of CDI and superior in reducing recurrence and achieving sustained clinical cure. Recurrence occurs in approximately 20% of patients treated with metronidazole or

Table 2.3. Management of *C. difficile* infection classified by severity.

CDI	Diagnosis	Treatment
Mild	WCC typically normal <3 stools of Type 5-7* per day	PO metronidazole 400-500mg tds for 10-14 days
Moderate	WCC 11-15 x 10^9/L 3-5 stools of Type 5-7* per day	PO metronidazole 400-500mg tds for 10-14 days
Severe	WCC >15 x 10^9/L or acutely rising creatinine (>50% above baseline) or temperature >38.5°C or evidence of severe colitis	PO vancomycin 125mg qds for 10-14 days
Life-threatening	Hypotension or partial or complete ileus or toxic megacolon or CT evidence of severe disease	PO vancomycin up to 500mg qds for 10-14 days

* Bristol Stool Chart

vancomycin and can be treated with the same initial agent. Subsequent recurrence should be treated with fidaxomicin because of the increased risk of further recurrences.

Faecal transplant rarely has adverse effects and causes resolution of CDI in 81% of patients. It is used as a last resort option, mainly due to practical and aesthetic concerns.

1. Public Health England. Updated guidance on the management and treatment of *Clostridium difficile* infection. London, UK: Public Health England, 2013.
2. Louie TJ, Miller MA, Mullane KM, *et al.* Fidaxomicin versus vancomycin for *Clostridium difficile* infection. *New Engl J Med* 2011; 364: 422-31.

82   A

Computed tomography imaging is frequently necessary in the critically ill to delineate pathology and guide prognosis. Often, contrast will be needed in patients who already have a degree of acute kidney injury. Various options to limit additional contrast-induced nephropathy have been explored, with variable supporting evidence.

Intravenous hydration pre-procedure has face validity and a number of small supporting trials. In addition, a recent study has compared the use of IV bicarbonate to normal saline for volume expansion and noted a degree of benefit with bicarbonate. A systematic review has led to generalised tentative recommendations to consider the use of intravenous bicarbonate as first-line hydration.

Intravenous N-acetyl cysteine (NAC) is not generally recommended due to a lack of supporting evidence and a risk of anaphylaxis. There are data to suggest that oral NAC given the day before and day after the procedure may confer some benefit at lower risk.

Fenoldopam (a D1 receptor agonist) and dopamine have no benefit in the prevention of contrast-induced nephropathy. High osmolal contrast agents make the likelihood of injury considerably higher and should be avoided where possible.

1.   Ozcan EE, Guneri S, Akdeniz B, *et al*. Sodium bicarbonate, N-acetylcysteine, and saline for prevention of radiocontrast-induced nephropathy. A comparison of 3 regimens for protecting contrast-induced nephropathy in patients undergoing coronary procedures. A single-centre prospective controlled trial. *Am Heart J* 2007; 154(3): 539.
2.   Hoste EA, De Waele JJ, Gevaert SA, *et al*. Sodium bicarbonate for prevention of contrast-induced acute kidney injury: a systematic review and meta-analysis. *Nephrol Dial Transplant* 2010; 25(3): 747.
3.   Trivedi H, Daram S, Szabo A, *et al*. High-dose N-acetylcysteine for the prevention of contrast-induced nephropathy. *Am J Med* 2009; 122(9): 874.e9.

83 D

The low cardiac output state with a high CVP and systemic vascular resistance index (SVRI), coupled with the signs of reverse pulsus paradoxus, suggest the diagnosis of cardiac tamponade. A rapid increase in pericardial fluid volume, typically seen with bleeding post-cardiac surgery, leads to a rapid rise in pressure within the pericardial cavity. Despite good drain placement, clots can form within the drains, disguising the amount of blood loss and leading to tamponade. A picture of decreased cardiac output with compensatory tachycardia and sympathetically-mediated vasoconstriction causes an increase in SVR to maintain MAP. Elevated CVP improves diastolic filling against raised intrapericardial pressure. Beck's triad of hypotension, elevated jugular venous pressure and muffled heart sounds are only present in a small number of patients with cardiac tamponade. Pulsus paradoxus (the exaggerated fall in blood pressure during the inspiratory phase of spontaneous ventilation) is more commonly seen. In a patient receiving positive pressure ventilation, reverse pulsus paradoxus can be seen. Pulsus paradoxus can also be seen in cases of severe asthma, pulmonary embolism and tension pneumothorax. Due to the oscillation of the heart within the pericardial sac, cyclical variations in QRS amplitude can be seen — electrical alternans. It is not unusual to see a normal chest X-ray with the development of acute tamponade.

1. World Federation of Societies of Anaesthesiologists. Odor P, Bailey A. Cardiac tamponade. Anaesthesia Tutorial of the Week 283, 18th March 2013. www.aagbi.org/education/educational-resources/tutorial-week (accessed 26th February 2015).
2. http://www.frca.co.uk/Documents/283%20Cardiac%20Tamponade%20.pdf (accessed 14th July 2014).

84 A

Burns patients should have airways secured early, as many of these patients have aggressive fluid management and consequently the airway may become oedematous and precarious if not secured early. All options are plausible to varying degrees but tracheal intubation is clearly the most appropriate given the severity of the inhalational injury described in the main stem of the question. While in some cases close observation may be reasonable, this patient has a significant burn injury and is certain to develop multi-organ failure and require mechanical ventilation in due course, so the best course of action is to secure the airway before the situation deteriorates. Awake fibreoptic intubation is likely to be very challenging in this patient with pain and distress, and is unlikely to be necessary in this case. While early intubation of burns patients is usually straightforward this should be performed by individuals with significant anaesthetic experience and with difficult airway equipment available.

1.   Bishop S, Maguire S. Anaesthesia and intensive care for major burns. *Contin Educ Anaesth Crit Care Pain* 2012; 12: 118-22.

85   B

This elderly patient is at high risk of developing respiratory complications due to his past medical history and the number of fractures sustained. With three or more rib fractures the rate of complications and mortality increase significantly. Good pain relief allows for proper ventilation, effective cough and adequate respiratory physiotherapy. Regional analgesic techniques, although invasive, in general, tend to be more effective than systemic opioids and cause less systemic side effects. It has been shown that thoracic epidural analgesia improves pain control, decreases rates of nosocomial pneumonia and mean ICU and hospital stay when compared with intravenous opiates. However, it does cause a significant increase in clinically significant hypotension.

The use of a paravertebral block can effectively be used for analgesia for fractured ribs and a catheter can be inserted for continuous analgesia. Due to the unilateral nature of the block achieved, hypotension is unusual and the analgesia achieved is comparable with that provided by a thoracic epidural. Intercostal blocks are an effective mode of analgesia for rib fractures and, again, a catheter can be inserted for continuous analgesia.

In the presence of clopidogrel (which irreversibly inhibits platelet function), the Association of Anaesthetists of Great Britain and Ireland (AAGBI) guidelines would recommend the discontinuation for at least 7 days prior to performing central neuraxial blockade (which would include paravertebral block). Intercostal blocks are regarded as peripheral nerve blocks with a much lower risk of clinically significant haemorrhage, and as such can be undertaken despite the use of clopidogrel. Entonox is a mixture of oxygen and nitrous oxide that provides immediate short-term pain relief, but it would exacerbate the pneumothorax and therefore not be useful in this situation. The benefit of changing oral to intravenous paracetamol is likely to be incremental.

For this patient a risk-benefit analysis should take place; intercostal blocks are the preferred option assuming the expertise exists and would need repeating at intervals. It may be that the risk of insertion of a paravertebral or epidural catheter would be outweighed by the potential benefits of good analgesia allowing secretion clearance, bearing in mind that this patient would not necessarily be a candidate for invasive ventilation in the event of further respiratory deterioration.

1. Gilart JF, Rodriguez HH, Vallina PM, *et al.* Guidelines for the diagnosis and treatment of thoracic traumatism. *Arch Bronconeumol* 2011; 47: 41-9.
2. Karmakar MK, Ho AM. Acute pain management of patients with multiple rib fractures. *J Trauma* 2003; 54(3): 615-25.
3. Tighe SQM, Greene MD, Rajadurai N. Paravertebral block. *Contin Educ Anaesth Crit Care Pain* 2010; 10(5): 133-7.
4. Association of Anaesthetists of Great Britain and Ireland, Obstetric Anaesthetists' Association and Regional Anaesthesia UK. Regional anaesthesia and patients with abnormalities of coagulation. *Anaesthesia* 2013; 68: 966-72.

86 C

Refeeding syndrome is defined as the clinical complications that occur as a result of fluid and electrolyte shifts during nutritional rehabilitation of significantly malnourished patients. It is a rare but potentially serious complication in the critically ill patient, often following the introduction of feed after a severe critical illness with catabolism.

It is characterised by hypophosphataemia, hypomagnesaemia and hypokalaemia. The pathogenesis of this focuses on depletion of body stores during critical illness and malnutrition, followed by the introduction of feed, insulin release and cellular uptake of remaining circulating electrolytes leading to extreme biochemical shifts and gross intravascular depletion. These shifts can result in clinical manifestations including cardiac dysrhythmias and dysfunction.

Management focuses on electrolyte replacement, reduction of feed quantity and careful monitoring. An open access review article has succinctly summarised the key features and NICE guidance recently.

1. Mehana HM, Moledina J, Travis J. Refeeding syndrome: what it is, and how to prevent and treat it. *Br Med J* 2008; 336(7659): 1495-8.

87 C

The signs found on examination suggest that this patient is suffering from hypovolaemic hypernatraemia. When hypovolaemia is present, urine should be maximally concentrated, with an osmolality of 800-1000mOsm/kg.

Diabetes insipidus (DI) is a disease in which large volumes of urine are excreted (polyuria in excess of 40-50ml/kg/24hr in the average adult) due to vasopressin deficiency (central DI) or vasopressin resistance (nephrogenic DI). After confirming polyuria, a 7-hour (or less) water deprivation test is usually sufficient to diagnose DI. If the polyuria is due to primary polydipsia then water deprivation will resolve the polyuria. Ongoing production of large volumes of inappropriately dilute urine suggests DI. Central and nephrogenic DI can then be differentiated by a desmopressin (DDAVP) challenge. An increase in the urine osmolality with DDAVP to greater than 750mOsm/kg diagnoses central DI. If the urine osmolality remains less than 300mOsm/kg then a diagnosis of nephrogenic DI can be made.

1. Adrogue HJ, Madias NE. Hypernatraemia. *New Engl J Med* 2000; 342(20): 1493-9.

2.   Di Iorgi N, Napoli F, Allegri AEM, *et al*. Diabetes insipidus - diagnosis and management. *Horm Res Paediatr* 2012; 77: 69-84.

88   E

Hypotension is a feature of life-threatening asthma, as opposed to merely acute severe asthma as defined in the British Thoracic Society guidelines, reflecting obstruction to venous return in the thoracic compartment due to gas trapping. The parameters for diagnosing an acute severe asthma attack are:

* Peak expiratory flow rate of between 30% and 50% of expected.
* Respiratory rate greater than 25 breaths/minute.
* Tachycardia: heart rate >110 beats per minute.
* Inability to complete sentences with one breath.

The parameters of life-threatening asthma are:

* Peak expiratory flow rate of <33% of best or predicted.
* Silent chest or poor respiratory effort.
* Exhaustion.
* Hypotension or arrhythmia.
* Bradycardia.
* Cyanosis or SpO_2 <92%.
* 'Normal' $PaCO_2$ (4.6-6kPa).

Near-fatal asthma is signified by a patient with a rising $PaCO_2$ requiring mechanical ventilation with raised inflation pressures.

1.   BTS/SIGN. British guideline on the management of asthma: a national clinical guideline 101. https://www.brit-thoracic.org.uk/document-library/clinical-information/asthma/btssign-guideline-on-the-management-of-asthma (accessed 1st June 2014).

89   C

Prevention of vasospasm and more importantly the delayed cerebral ischaemia (DCI) that can result remains challenging. Aspects to consider include proactive monitoring of vasospasm versus management of clinically relevant DCI, the concept of prophylaxis against actual treatment of DCI once established and the risk benefit profile of rescue therapy.

International consensus guidelines have been produced on the management of subarachnoid haemorrhage within the last 2 years, which cover the evidence related to this troublesome issue. Whilst enteral nimodipine is supported by several large systematic reviews and meta-analyses, there are no data to support the use of intravenous calcium channel blockers to treat vasospasm and their use can significantly impinge on cerebral perfusion pressure. Hypervolaemia and haemodilution have been largely discredited as targets of therapy, with the frequent development of pulmonary oedema and subsequent hypoxia leading to unacceptable risk in the brain-injured patient. Induced hypertension is thought to be the key aspect responsible for the previous success of triple-H therapy and as such continues to be recommended for the management of DCI.

Statins have shown promise, but recent meta-analysis would suggest that while they display a trend towards improved outcome, they show no significant benefit in the prevention or treatment of DCI.

1.   Sander Connolly E, Rabinstein AA, Carhuapoma JR, *et al*. Guidelines for the management of subarachnoid haemorrhage. *Stroke* 2012; 43: 1711-37.
2.   Harrigan M. Hypertension may be the most important component of hyperdynamic therapy in cerebral vasospasm. *Crit Care* 2010; 14: 151.
3.   Kramer AH, Fletcher JJ. Statins in the management of patients with aneurysmal subarachnoid haemorrhage: a systematic review and meta-analysis. *Neurocrit Care* 2010; 12(2): 285-96.

90   B

The causes of acute kidney injury (AKI) can be divided into three categories: pre-renal, intrinsic renal, and post-renal. This patient has risk factors for all three categories but the cause can be differentiated using fractional excretion of sodium, urine and serum osmolalities, urinalysis and imaging modalities. Fractional excretion of sodium (FeNa) is calculated as follows:

([Urinary Na^+ / serum Na^+] / [urinary creatinine/serum creatinine] x 100)

It is based on the premise that intact tubules will reabsorb sodium in the pre-renal setting, whereas injured tubules occurring with acute tubular necrosis (ATN) will not. Values <1% suggest a pre-renal cause, >3% suggests ATN. Urinalysis can be used to evaluate the cause of AKI. Bland sediment and hyaline casts are consistent with pre-renal AKI. The presence of renal tubular epithelial cells, coarse granular casts and renal tubular epithelial cell casts are evidence for ATN. Visualisation of red blood cell casts in the urine sediment is indicative of glomerulonephritis. In cases of acute interstitial nephritis, eosinophils and white blood cell casts are seen.

The high fractional excretion of sodium and visualisation of coarse granular casts and renal tubular epithelial cell casts suggest a diagnosis of acute tubular necrosis. Nephrotoxins should be eliminated and treatment for the underlying cause should be instigated.

1. Rahman M, Shad F, Smith MC. Acute kidney injury: a guide to diagnosis and management. *Am Fam Physician* 2012; 86(7): 631-9.
2. Perazella MA, Coca SG. Traditional urinary biomarkers in the assessment of hospital-acquired AKI. *Clin J Am Soc Nephrol* 2012; 7: 167-74.

Multiple True False (MTF) questions — select true or false for each of the five stems.

1 Regarding non-invasive ventilation (NIV) in criticaly ill patients:

a. It has a clear mortality benefit in patients with Type I respiratory failure due to chronic obstructive pulmonary disease (COPD) compared with standard medical therapy.
b. It is contraindicated in patients with thoracic wall deformities.
c. It is an effective treatment for severe community-acquired pneumonia.
d. It should be first-line therapy for asthmatic patients with worsening respiratory acidosis.
e. It is effective rescue therapy following failed extubation.

2 In a patient currently receiving cytotoxic chemotherapy with a fever:

a. A neutrophil count of less than 1 x 10^9/L confirms the diagnosis of neutropaenia.
b. Empirical combination therapy with piperacillin/tazobactam and aminoglycoside cover is recommended as first line in national guidance.
c. Indwelling catheters should be removed and sent for microbiological assessment during initial management.
d. Granulocyte colony-stimulating factor (G-CSF) should be administered within the first 48 hours.
e. Patients with indwelling central venous access devices should receive glycopeptide antibiotics within 48 hours of presentation.

3 Regarding the anterior triangle of the neck:

a.   It is bounded anteriorly by the sternocleidomastoid muscle.
b.   The trachea lies deep to the anterior triangle.
c.   It contains the vagus nerve.
d.   Skin is punctured within the anterior triangle when using a landmark technique for internal jugular central venous access.
e.   The common carotid artery can be palpated in the anterior triangle at the inferior border of the mandible.

4 Causes of hypercalcaemia include:

a.   Loop diuretics.
b.   Multiple endocrine neoplasia (MEN) Type IIb.
c.   Theophylline toxicity.
d.   Hyperthyroidism.
e.   Immobilisation.

5 With regard to glycaemic control in the critically ill patient:

a.   The risk of mortality increases with variable glycaemic control in a 'dose-dependent' manner.
b.   The VISEP (Efficacy of Volume Substitution and Insulin Therapy in Severe Sepsis) study supports the use of intensive insulin therapy and tight glycaemic control to reduce mortality and sequential organ failure.
c.   The NICE SUGAR (Normoglycemia in Intensive Care Evaluation and Surviving Using Glucose Algorithm Regulation) study supports the use of intensive insulin therapy and tight glycaemic control to reduce mortality and sequential organ failure.
d.   Intensive insulin control within a clinical trial environment does not increase the likelihood of acute hypoglycaemic events.
e.   The standard target for conventional glucose control in adult critical care is 4-8mmol/L.

6 Regarding vascular access during cardiopulmonary resuscitation (CPR):

a. If intravenous access cannot be secured within the first 2 minutes of CPR, intraosseous access should be considered.
b. Peripherally injected drugs should be flushed with at least 20ml of fluid.
c. Drug doses should be doubled if delivered via the intraosseous route.
d. Tracheal drug administration is no longer recommended.
e. Flow rates are higher when intraosseous access is secured in the tibia than the humerus.

7 Regarding the use of a laryngeal mask airway (LMA):

a. It can be easily inserted without neuromuscular blockade.
b. Is highly effective in maintaining a patent airway.
c. It can be used with positive pressure ventilation.
d. Is contraindicated with muscle relaxants.
e. Is safe to use with a full stomach.

8 Evidence-based rescue strategies shown to reduce mortality in severe acute respiratory distress syndrome (ARDS) include the following:

a. Paralysis using non-depolarising muscle relaxants.
b. Therapeutic hypothermia.
c. High-frequency oscillatory ventilation.
d. Airway pressure release ventilation.
e. Inhaled nitric oxide.

9 Life-threatening chest injuries which should be addressed in the primary survey according to Advanced Trauma Life Support (ATLS) guidelines include:

a. Oesophageal rupture.
b. Cardiac tamponade.
c. Traumatic aortic disruption.
d. Traumatic diaphragmatic injury.
e. Open pneumothorax.

10 A patient is bleeding postoperatively. His platelet count is now 90mmol/L (previously 140mmol/L). The ICU team organise a thromboelastogram (TEG®) as part of the work-up. The following apply to this test:

a. The TEG® is suitable for near-patient testing.
b. The reaction time (R-time) represents the speed of solid clot formation.
c. The α-angle has a normal value of 60-70°.
d. The K (clot formation) time reflects the contribution of fibrinogen, platelets and intrinsic clotting factors to the clotting process.
e. The maximum amplitude (MA) is increased in thrombocytopaenia.

11 With regard to statistics and evidence-based medicine:

a. An odds ratio is equivalent to a risk ratio.
b. Absolute risk reduction (ARR) is the only value required to calculate the number needed to treat (NNT).
c. A Type I error reflects a false-negative result.
d. A funnel plot is used to represent heterogeneity within a systematic review.
e. An intention to treat analysis aims to assess the efficacy of a treatment, rather than its effectiveness.

12 The following are true of trauma scoring systems:

a. An Abbreviated Injury Scale (AIS) score of 1 denotes an unsurvivable injury.
b. The maximum value obtainable for the Injury Severity Score (ISS) is 50.
c. The Revised Trauma Score (RTS) is an anatomical scoring system.
d. The Trauma Injury Severity Score (TRISS) uses the ISS, AIS and the patient's age to determine a probability of survival.
e. Different values are calculated for blunt and penetrating injuries using the Injury Severity Score.

13 A 56-year-old male is intubated, sedated and ventilated for respiratory decompensation. He has a large left pleural effusion which is aspirated under ultrasound guidance. The protein level of the aspirate is 24g/L. Which of the following apply to pleural effusions?:

a. A pleural protein of 24g/L is suggestive of an exudate.
b. Nephrotic syndrome is a cause of a transudate.
c. Measurement of lactate dehydrogenase is useful to distinguish exudative from transudative pleural effusions.
d. Haemorrhagic pleural fluids are pathognomonic of malignancy.
e. A low pleural fluid glucose content would be consistent with infection or malignancy.

14 In paediatric advanced life support, the following formulae are relevant and considered accurate:

a. Energy required for DC cardioversion is 2J/kg.
b. The weight of a 3-year-old child can be calculated using the formula (2 x age in years)+8.
c. Amiodarone for refractory ventricular tachycardia (VT) is dosed at 5mg/kg.
d. Ceftriaxone for meningococcal septicaemia is dosed at 80mg/kg.
e. The internal diameter of a suitable endotracheal tube is calculated by age/2 + 4.

Paper 3 Questions

223

15 Regarding the prevention of healthcare-associated infections in the critical care setting:

a. Effective hand washing requires rubbing hands together for a minimum of 60 seconds, once liquid soap or an antimicrobial preparation has been applied.
b. Alcohol-based hand rubs are not suitable for spore-forming bacteria.
c. After performing a procedure, gowns should be removed before gloves to minimise the risk of cross-contamination.
d. Bacteriuria is largely preventable if urinary catheterisation is performed with a strict aseptic technique.
e. Dressings on central venous catheters (CVCs) should be changed at a minimum every 3 days.

16 A man is admitted with rapidly progressive cellulitis. He is a diabetic and has renal failure. He is in septic shock. A diagnosis of necrotising fasciitis (NF) is considered. Regarding this condition:

a. Skin changes typically precede the pain in NF.
b. It is most commonly polymicrobial.
c. Intravenous antibiotic therapy is the mainstay of treatment.
d. Muscle involvement is required for the diagnosis to be made.
e. It is classified according to location of the disease.

17 Regarding a trauma patient with a potential cervical spine injury:

a. Attempts to clinically clear the spine without radiology should not be made in patients over 65 years of age.
b. The patient should have three plain view cervical radiographs as first-line imaging.
c. Following a normal CT of the cervical spine, the chance of unstable injury requiring neurosurgical intervention or ongoing immobilisation is less than 1%.

d.   Three-point immobilisation is supported by level I evidence to improve outcome.

e.   Aspen collars are preferred to hard collars for soft tissue neck injury.

18 Regarding the discriminatory power of tests and scoring systems:

a.   A false-positive means the patient does not have the disease and the test is negative.

b.   The specificity of a test is calculated by the (number of true negatives) divided by the (number of true negatives plus the number of false positives).

c.   The positive predictive value of a test is influenced by the prevalence of the disease.

d.   A receiver operator characteristic (ROC) curve plots sensitivity against specificity.

e.   The larger the area under the ROC curve, the higher the discriminatory power of the test.

19 Regarding hypertrophic cardiomyopathy (HCM):

a.   It is the most common cause of spontaneous cardiac arrest in young athletes.

b.   It is characterised by severe left ventricular hypertrophy in association with aortic stenosis.

c.   The most common echocardiographic characteristic is systolic anterior motion of the anterior aortic valve leaflet with left ventricular outflow obstruction.

d.   β-blockers are relatively contraindicated.

e.   There is an association between hypertrophic cardiomyopathy and Wolff-Parkinson-White syndrome.

20 Regarding a patient with a penetrating neck injury:

a.   The platysma may or may not be breached.
b.   Multidetector CT imaging is very sensitive for the detection of clinically significant vascular injury.
c.   The patient should be immediately immobilised in a hard collar.
d.   Dysphonia is an indication for urgent surgical exploration.
e.   A negative CT effectively excludes aerodigestive tract injury.

21 The following ECG features support a diagnosis of right ventricular hypertrophy:

a.   Axis deviation of +110° or more.
b.   R-wave 8mm tall in V1.
c.   R/S ratio <1 in lead V5 or V6.
d.   Bifid P-waves.
e.   ST depression/T-wave inversion in V5-6.

22 Which of the following are recommended as drugs to terminate status epilepticus in the adult patient according to NICE guidelines?

a.   Sodium valproate.
b.   Suxamethonium.
c.   Ketamine.
d.   Propofol.
e.   Lorazepam.

23 The following are validated tools in predicting outcome post-cardiac arrest:

a. N20 somatosensory evoked potential from the median nerve.
b. Glasgow Coma Scale (GCS) at 24 hours.
c. Myoclonic status epilepticus.
d. CT brain consistent with hypoxic brain injury.
e. Fixed dilated pupils on admission to the intensive care unit.

24 Regarding drug resistance and the use of antimicrobials in critical care:

a. Multidrug resistance (MDR) is defined as acquired non-susceptibility to at least one agent in five or more antimicrobial categories.
b. Resistant strains of *Enterococcus* carry the Panton-Valentine leukocidin virulence factor.
c. Methicillin-resistant *Staphylococcus aureus* (MRSA) can be treated with meropenem.
d. Tigecycline has activity against MRSA.
e. Linezolid is highly effective when given orally.

25 A man is admitted to your ICU with acute liver failure. The following criteria must be met to fulfil a diagnosis of acute liver failure:

a. Illness duration <28 days.
b. Presence of chronic liver disease.
c. Jaundice.
d. Coagulopathy with an INR >1.5.
e. Encephalopathy.

26 The following statements are true regarding the evidential base for care of the cardiac arrest patient following return of spontaneous circulation:

a. Level I evidence supports the use of early angiography in all patients with suspected cardiac aetiology.
b. Hyperoxia has been shown to worsen outcomes in a randomised controlled trial.
c. Targeted temperature management has been demonstrated to significantly improve outcomes compared to no temperature control.
d. Avoidance of hyperglycaemia >10mmol/L is supported by consensus recommendation.
e. Initiation of β-blockade is supported by level II evidence.

27 Regarding the principles and practical aspects of pulse oximetry:

a. Pulse oximetry uses three lights of different absorption spectra to measure blood oxygen saturations.
b. Oximeters are inaccurate at a saturation of <80%.
c. A pulse oximeter can distinguish between carboxyhaemoglobin and oxyhaemoglobin.
d. Oxyhaemoglobin is overestimated when elevated levels of methaemoglobin are present.
e. Severe jaundice will not alter oximetry readings.

28 The following variables are used in the calculation of the Acute Physiology and Chronic Health Evaluation (APACHE) II score:

a. Age.
b. Systolic blood pressure.
c. Temperature.
d. Serum calcium.
e. Gender.

29 The following are causes of a raised anion gap metabolic acidosis:

a. Renal failure.
b. Lactic acidosis.
c. Externally draining pancreatic fistula.
d. Excessive infusion of normal saline.
e. Urinary diversion.

30 The following statements are true concerning the checking of medical device placement with a chest X-ray:

a. A chest X-ray confirms satisfactory placement of a tracheostomy tube.
b. The tip of a central venous catheter seen on chest X-ray at the level of the carina suggests satisfactory placement.
c. In adults the tip of an endotracheal tube should be 5-6cm above the carina.
d. A nasogastric tube should be seen to cross the diaphragm in the midline.
e. A chest radiograph must be performed to confirm correct tracheostomy placement.

31 A 38-year-old woman is admitted with severe urosepsis. Her blood pressure is 89/50mmHg, heart rate is 110 beats per minute and temperature is 39.9°C. Her initial lactate is 5.9mmol/L. She has received 3L of 0.9% saline as part of her fluid resuscitation. This lactate has reduced to 3.9mmol/L.

a.   Lactate is cleared from the blood mainly by skeletal muscle.
b.   She is likely to have a Type A lactic acidosis.
c.   She is likely to have a normal anion gap.
d.   Normal subjects produce 15-20mmol of lactic acid per day.
e.   Lactic acid is produced from the metabolism of lactate dehydrogenase.

32 Regarding the potential organ donor patient:

a.   Warm ischaemic time is reduced in donation after cardiac death (DCD) cases, compared to donation after brainstem death (DBD).
b.   DCD patients cannot donate lungs.
c.   Controlled DCD patients are Maastricht category III and IV.
d.   Organ retrieval should be commenced immediately following the onset of asystole in DCD donors.
e.   A nurse with a specialist role in organ donation is an appropriate person to make the initial approach to the family.

33 Regarding the principles of invasive blood pressure monitoring:

a.   The risk of thrombus formation is greater with a wide-bore arterial cannula.
b.   The flush system infuses continuously at about 20-30ml/hr.
c.   The addition of extra tubing and three-way-taps to the system cause an increase in damping.
d.   Overdamping has no effect on the reading of mean arterial pressure.

e. The transducer must be at the level of the heart when the system is zeroed.

34 A 49-year-old woman is admitted with sepsis. As part of her examination, the ICU doctor notices a hot swollen right knee joint. On further questioning the patient complains of pain in all range of movements. She denies any trauma and has no history of previous joint problems. She is otherwise fit and well and is taking no regular medications. She is pyrexial (38.1°C) and has an erythrocyte sedimentation rate (ESR) of 80mm/hr. A diagnosis of possible septic arthritis is made. Regarding this diagnosis:

a. A negative Gram stain of the joint fluid aspirate makes the diagnosis unlikely.
b. Plain X-ray of the affected joint is often non-diagnostic.
c. An elevated C-reactive protein (CRP) has a high positive predictive value for septic arthritis.
d. A positive Gram stain has a very high positive predictive value for septic arthritis.
e. Diagnostic aspiration should be performed within 2 hours of suspecting the diagnosis.

35 The following preconditions must be met before brainstem death testing can be undertaken on the intensive care unit:

a. pH 7.35 to 7.45.
b. Core temperature >34°C.
c. Serum potassium >2mmol/L.
d. Mean arterial pressure consistently >60mmHg.
e. Serum sodium >125mmol/L.

Paper 3 Questions

36 The following are risk factors for the development of a pulmonary embolism:

a. Heparin-induced thrombocytopaenia.
b. General anaesthesia for >30 minutes.
c. Antiphospholipid antibodies.
d. Immune thrombocytopaenia.
e. Obesity.

37 Regarding serotonin syndrome (SS):

a. Cyproheptadine is a precipitating cause.
b. It has no extrapyramidal signs.
c. Onset is typically over a period of several days.
d. Ondansetron is a method of treatment.
e. The presence of autonomic instability should prompt a search for an alternative diagnosis.

38 With regard to thromboelastography (TEG®):

a. R-time represents time to clot initiation.
b. MA represents mean acceleration, or the speed at which fibrin build-up and cross-linking occurs ('the thrombin burst').
c. K-time represents the time to achieve a certain level of clot strength.
d. Enhanced fibrinolysis is represented visually by a coming together at baseline of the upper and lower trace several minutes into the recording.
e. There is level I evidence to support its use in guiding product replacement for the major trauma patient.

39 Regarding the management of massive haemorrhage:

a. Protamine sulphate should be considered for patients anticoagulated with low-molecular-weight heparin (LMWH).
b. In the acutely bleeding patient, a minimum target platelet count of 150 x 10⁹/L is appropriate.
c. Tranexamic acid has a mortality benefit if given within 12 hours of the traumatic event.
d. In an emergency, group O Rh positive blood can be safely transfused if the patient's blood group is not known.
e. Following major haemorrhage pharmacological thromboprophylaxis should normally be omitted for 5-7 days.

40 A 67-year-old woman is admitted after an accidental fall and sustains a massive subdural haematoma. She is taken to theatre as an emergency and undergoes evacuation of the haematoma. She remains ventilated on the intensive care unit. Seven days after the operation she desaturates and multiple pulmonary emboli are demonstrated on a contrast computed tomography pulmonary angiogram (CTPA). Consideration is given to siting a vena cava filter. Regarding this treatment:

a. Vena cava filters improve survival in patients with pulmonary embolism and contraindications to anticoagulation.
b. Consensus guidelines recommend prophylactic vena cava filter placement on admission to the ICU for patients such as this.
c. Once sited the filter cannot be removed.
d. The vena cava filter reduces the incidence of further pulmonary emboli.
e. The presence of a vena cava filter would preclude future magnetic resonance imaging in this lady.

41 When diagnosing death:

a. Death after cardiorespiratory arrest can be diagnosed without attempting to auscultate heart sounds or palpate a pulse.
b. The individual should be observed by the person responsible for confirming death for a minimum of 3 minutes to establish irreversible cardiorespiratory arrest has occurred.
c. The patient's temperature should be greater than 35.5°C before brainstem death testing is performed.
d. Serum potassium levels must be >2mmol/L before brainstem testing can be performed.
e. In cases of high spinal cord injury, ancillary tests must be performed to diagnose brainstem death.

42 In the diagnosis and management of hyponatraemia:

a. Acute hyponatraemia is hyponatraemia that is documented to exist for less than 24 hours.
b. Syndrome of inappropriate antidiuretic hormone secretion (SIADH) causes a hypotonic hyponatraemia with normal extracellular fluid volume.
c. The increase in sodium concentration during the first 24 hours should be limited to 1mmol/L/hr.
d. In a patient with severe symptoms of hyponatraemia, rapid administration of 3% hypertonic saline is recommended.
e. Following correction of hyponatraemia, if symptoms fail to resolve immediately they should not be attributed to the electrolyte disturbance.

43 Regarding intensive care unit delirium, which of the following statements are true?

a. ICU delirium occurs in 30-45% of ICU patients.
b. It is commonly over-diagnosed.

c. The hyperactive form is the most common.
d. The CAM-ICU test requires knowledge of the patient's sedation score.
e. Benzodiazepines are the first-line treatment.

44 In a patient with a percutaneous tracheostomy that is potentially blocked:

a. Oxygen should be applied to the face and tracheostomy immediately.
b. Inner tubes should be left in to facilitate connection to a breathing circuit.
c. The cuff should be deflated prior to attempting to pass a suction catheter.
d. The tracheostomy tube should not be removed if difficult endotracheal intubation is predicted.
e. A paediatric face mask applied to the stoma can be used as a primary emergency oxygenation strategy.

45 Regarding the diagnosis and management of pulmonary hypertension:

a. Patients with pulmonary hypertension most commonly present with peripheral oedema.
b. Pulmonary hypertension can be formally diagnosed using echocardiography.
c. Sleep disordered breathing is a recognised cause of pulmonary hypertension.
d. Treatment options include high-dose calcium channel blockade.
e. Bosentan lowers pulmonary vascular resistance by inhibiting phosphodiesterase Type 5.

46 The following results of the cerebrospinal fluid (CSF) analysis are characteristic in Guillain-Barré syndrome (GBS):

a. Monoclonal bands.
b. Protein <0.5g/L.
c. CSF glucose >2/3 of plasma glucose.
d. Lymphocytosis.
e. Opening pressure of 35cm H_2O.

47 With regard to the practice of selective decontamination of the digestive tract (SDD):

a. Drugs used in the regime include polymyxin, amphotericin and tobramycin.
b. There is level I evidence that the intervention reduces the risk of ventilator-associated pneumonia (VAP).
c. There is good evidence to suggest increased rates of antibiotic resistance with the intervention.
d. The SUDDICU (Selective Decontamination of the Digestive tract in critically ill patients treated in Intensive Care Units) trial demonstrated a reduction in all-cause mortality with the intervention.
e. Increased rates of *Clostridium difficile* are a common problem.

48 Regarding the pathophysiology of acquired and hereditary bleeding disorders:

a. Von Willebrand Factor promotes the binding of platelets to the subendothelium.
b. In acquired haemophilia, coagulation in a laboratory sample will normalise when fresh frozen plasma is added to the sample.
c. Heparin-induced thrombocytopaenia is caused by an antibody to platelet GP Ia receptors.

d.   Glanzmann thrombasthenia is an acquired disorder of platelet function.
e.   Vasopressin can be used to reduce the bleeding time in von Willebrand disease.

49 Regarding the Sengstaken-Blakemore tube and its use in upper gastrointestinal variceal haemorrhage:

a.   It has four ports.
b.   Must be stored at 4°C.
c.   Requires insertion via the oral route.
d.   Rebleeding is common after deflation of the gastric balloon.
e.   The tube should be removed within 12 hours of insertion to prevent pressure necrosis.

50 With regard to thrombolysis in the management of submassive and massive pulmonary embolism, which of the following statements are correct?

a.   Right ventricular dysfunction on echo is a relative contraindication to thrombolysis.
b.   Elderly patients are significantly more likely to have a major bleed with thrombolysis for pulmonary embolism compared with anticoagulation only.
c.   Thrombolysis for pulmonary embolism requires an interventional radiologist for delivery.
d.   There is no evidence for a mortality benefit of thrombolysis compared with therapeutic anticoagulation alone.
e.   There are no large randomised controlled trials studying thrombolysis in this patient group.

51 Regarding the diagnosis and management of acute severe pancreatitis:

a. Serum amylase remains within the normal range in approximately a third of patients with acute pancreatitis.
b. All patients with a suspected diagnosis of acute pancreatitis should undergo a CT or MRI scan to assess severity.
c. Organ failure must be present for a diagnosis of severe acute pancreatitis to be made.
d. If necrosis of the pancreas is seen on CT, then antibiotics should be commenced to prevent infection of sterile pancreatic necrosis.
e. In severe acute pancreatitis, parenteral feeding is recommended to prevent infectious complications.

52 A 56-year-old man is admitted with a spontaneous pneumothorax. Aspiration has been attempted without success. He needs a chest drain inserting. Which of the following form part of the anatomical border of the 'safe triangle'?

a. Anterior border of the latissimus dorsi muscle.
b. Medial border of the latissimus dorsi muscle.
c. Lateral border of the pectoralis major muscle.
d. A line inferior to the horizontal level of the nipple.
e. An apex below the axilla.

53 Regarding the management of acute ST-elevation myocardial infarction (STEMI):

a. Angiography with follow-on percutaneous coronary intervention (PCI) is the preferred reperfusion strategy for people with acute STEMI if it can be delivered within 90 minutes of the time when fibrinolysis could have been given.

b. Angiography with follow-on percutaneous coronary intervention should only be performed if the patient presents within 12 hours of onset of symptoms.

c. Patients with a Glasgow Coma Score of 8 or less should not undergo reperfusion therapy.

d. During percutaneous coronary intervention all patients should receive a parenteral anticoagulant.

e. In the year following a STEMI, the risk of suffering another myocardial infarction is statistically less if a patient is treated with ticagrelor rather than clopidogrel.

54 Which of the following are causes of raised pulmonary artery occlusion pressure (PAOP)?

a. Right ventricular failure.
b. Aortic stenosis.
c. Mitral regurgitation.
d. Hypovolaemia.
e. Mitral stenosis.

55 A 7-year-old boy is taken from a house fire to the emergency department of his local hospital with burns to the back of his head, neck and back (approximately 21% body surface area). They are assessed by a plastic surgeon as involving the epidermis and the entire papillary dermis down to the reticular dermis. He weighs 24kg. Which of the following statements are true?

a. His percentage burns can be estimated using the 'rule of nines'.
b. His burns are deep partial thickness.
c. He should be managed in a burns centre.
d. During the first 8 hours from time of injury he should be given approximately 1L of intravenous fluid resuscitation.
e. If his carboxyhemoglobin level exceeds 5%, he should be transferred to a facility capable of delivering hyperbaric oxygen therapy.

56 Regarding the measurement of temperature on the intensive care unit:

a. Temperature measured in the upper third of the oesophagus correlates well with core temperature.

b. The pulmonary artery catheter uses a thermistor to measure temperature.

c. Tympanic thermometers measure the frequency of infrared light emitted by the tympanic membrane.

d. Thermometers using heat-sensitive chemical dots have a faster reaction time than mercury thermometers.

e. A low urinary flow rate improves the accuracy in measuring core body temperature using a bladder thermometer.

57 Which of the following are common features of 3, 4-methylene-dioxymethamphetamine (MDMA or ecstasy) toxicity?

a. Hepatotoxcity.
b. Hypernatraemia.
c. Hypothermia.
d. Postural hypotension.
e. Rhabdomyolysis.

58 The following are independent variables in Stewart's acid-base hypothesis:

a. pCO_2.
b. HCO_3^-.
c. ATOT.
d. $Log^{10}[H^+]$.
e. Strong ion difference (SID).

59 In the critically ill patient under consideration for red cell transfusion:

a. Using a restrictive transfusion trigger of 7g/dL has not been shown to confer a mortality benefit, when compared to a trigger of 9g/dL.
b. Recombinant erythropoietin is an effective alternative to blood transfusion in the Jehovah's Witness patient with acute blood loss.
c. There is level I evidence to suggest that patients with symptomatic coronary artery disease should be transfused to a Hb >10g/dL.
d. Patients with non-exsanguinating acute upper GI bleeding should be transfused to a restrictive trigger of >7g/dL only, to reduce the risk of rebleeding.
e. There is level I evidence to support restrictive transfusion in stable paediatric patients in a critical care environment.

60 Regarding the physiology of the lungs during mechanical ventilation:

a. Normal static lung compliance is 50-100ml/cmH$_2$O.
b. Plateau pressure = $P_{compliance}$ - $P_{resistance}$.
c. Volume-controlled ventilation produces a square inspiratory flow pattern.
d. CO$_2$ elimination is proportional to minute volume.
e. Ventilation is greater at the lung bases in healthy spontaneously breathing individuals.

Single best answer questions — select ONE answer from the five choices

61 A 23-year-old is anaesthetised for an emergency appendicectomy and undergoes a rapid sequence induction with thiopentone and suxamethonium. The anaesthetist is concerned as the patient's temperature is noted to be 38.5°C 20 minutes into the operation raising the possibility of malignant hyperthermia (MH). Which of the following is the most reliable early indicator of malignant hyperthermia?

a.   Metabolic alkalosis on arterial blood gas.
b.   Hyperthermia.
c.   Progressive hypercarbia.
d.   Myoglobinuria.
e.   Use of suxamethonium.

62 A 24-year-old male with traumatic brain injury has been declared brainstem dead on your ICU this morning. He was on the organ donor register and his family has been consulted. They, in agreement with the medical team, are keen to proceed to donation after brainstem death. Whilst awaiting the transplant team he becomes cardiovascularly unstable with a blood pressure of 90/30mmHg (MAP 50mmHg). He has crystalloid fluid running through a peripheral IV line and is currently 3L positive on cumulative balance. He has no central access. Which is the most appropriate next step?

a.   Commence him on a peripheral metaraminol infusion.
b.   Contact the transplant team to expedite surgery.
c.   Abandon plans for organ donation and stop mechanical ventilation.

d. Site a central venous catheter and commence him on low-dose vasopressin.

e. Prescribe a further fluid bolus of 500ml 4.5% human albumin solution.

63 An 82-year-old female is admitted with a 2-hour history of severe shortness of breath. Past medical history includes asthma, ischaemic heart disease and hypertension. Examination reveals pulmonary oedema, which is confirmed by the chest X-ray. An ECG shows atrial fibrillation with a ventricular rate of 155 beats per minute and a QTc of 400ms. She has no history of atrial fibrillation. What should be the first line of management?

a. Amiodarone.
b. Replacement of magnesium and potassium.
c. Diuretics.
d. Synchronised DC shock.
e. Esmolol infusion.

64 A 56-year-old male with a history of hypertension is taken unwell with chest pain and collapse. He vomits several times in the ambulance on the way to the emergency department. On examination he is pale and sweaty with chest pain radiating through to his back. He has a BP of 215/120mmHg in the left arm and a weaker right radial pulse. The most likely diagnosis is:

a. Type 1 myocardial infarction.
b. Acute rupture of the mitral valve.
c. Paradoxical embolism.
d. Boerhaave's syndrome.
e. Dissecting aortic aneurysm.

65 A 30-year-old polytrauma patient is admitted to your district general intensive care unit in the night. He has sustained significant head injuries alongside facial fractures and was intubated in the emergency department. The CT reports a right-sided subdural collection with contrecoup contusions, right retro-orbital haematoma and right-sided zygomatic arch, orbital roof and frontal sinus fractures. He has no neck or trunk injuries. There is no intracranial pressure monitoring in place. On arrival to the unit you notice that his right eye is proptosed with injected conjunctivae. He remains deeply sedated and paralysed. Which of the following is the most suitable next step?

a.   Lateral canthotomy.
b.   Ocular massage with Honan balloon.
c.   Urgent neurosurgical decompression.
d.   Sonographic optic nerve sheath evaluation.
e.   Adjust minute ventilation to low-normal $PaCO_2$.

66 A 34-year-old HIV-positive man is admitted with a 4-day history of headache, lethargy and photophobia. On examination he is found to have a positive Kernig's sign, neck stiffness and pyrexia. After a normal CT of the head, a lumbar puncture is performed. CSF analysis shows a protein of 1.1g/L, a glucose of 1.6mmol/L, a WCC of 250/mm^3 (mainly mononuclear), a negative Gram stain and negative India ink stain. (His blood sugar level is measured at 6.3mmol/L). The most likely diagnosis is:

a.   Cryptococcal meningitis.
b.   Viral meningitis.
c.   Toxoplasmosis encephalitis.

d.   TB meningitis.
e.   Bacterial meningitis.

67 A 28-year-old presents 30 weeks into her second pregnancy feeling unwell, with backache, fever and rigors. She has a temperature of 39.5°C. Urinalysis shows leucocytes ++ and protein +++. Her blood pressure is 80/50mmHg, heart rate is 110 beats per minute and her ECG shows a sinus tachycardia. Which action is most appropriate?

a.   Admit to critical care and administer intravenous broad-spectrum antibiotics immediately.
b.   Arrange urgent ultrasound of the renal tract.
c.   Oral antibiotics and admission to the antenatal unit.
d.   Urgent Caesarean section.
e.   Send a urine sample for microbiological assessment and start antibiotics based on white cell count and bacteriology.

68 A 55-year-old drug user is admitted to the unit after being found semi-conscious at home in an awkward position. He has clinical evidence of compartment syndrome to the left leg and is taken to theatre for fasciotomy. On transfer to the intensive care unit, the anaesthetist reports his latest blood gas to show a pH of 7.23, base excess -12 and potassium of 6.1mmol/L. His potassium was 4.4mmol/L in the emergency department. Blood pressure is currently 100/40mmHg unsupported. Urine output has been poor at approximately 10-15ml/hr since admission. He has had a total of 5L crystalloid since admission 16 hours earlier. CVP currently reads at 6mmHg. What is the most appropriate next management step?

a.   Initiation of continuous venovenous haemofiltration.
b.   Alkalinisation of the urine with sodium bicarbonate.
c.   Further fluid loading until the CVP is greater than 10mmHg.
d.   Noradrenaline infusion titrating to a MAP of 70-80mmHg.
e.   Intravenous mannitol 0.5-1g/kg ideal body weight.

69 During early rhabdomyolysis all of the features listed are typical EXCEPT:

a.   Raised creatine kinase.
b.   Red cell casts on urine microscopy.
c.   Hypocalcaemia.
d.   Blood +++ on urinalysis.
e.   Hyperphosphataemia.

70 A patient is found to have a corrected calcium of 3.20mmol/L. He is confused. He is given 3L of 0.9% saline over 24 hours. His corrected calcium is rechecked after 24 hours and is 3.10mmol/L. His mucous membranes are moist. His parathyroid hormone (PTH) level is suppressed. He is still confused. Which of the following is the most appropriate next step in his management?

a.   No further treatment required and continue to monitor his calcium levels.
b.   Continue with intravenous 0.9% saline of 3-4L/day.
c.   Intravenous bisphosphonate.
d.   Haemodialysis.
e.   Loop diuretic therapy.

71 A patient is transferred to the intensive care unit following a two-stage Ivor Lewis oesophagectomy. His background history includes peptic ulcer disease and chronic kidney disease (CKD) Stage 2. The note from the anaesthetist comments on difficulties with the epidural pre-operatively and records a patchy block only. On arrival, he has a bupivacaine infusion running at 15ml/hr through the epidural (which has been recently topped up) in addition to a patient-controlled analgesia system with fentanyl at 20μg/5 min availability. He is alert and orientated but continues to complain of severe pain when stimulated and has difficulty coughing. Blood pressure is currently 95/45mmHg supported by noradrenaline at 6ml/hr of 4mg in 50ml. Which of the following options (administered systemically) would be the best choice for adjuvant analgesia?

a. Ketamine.
b. Pregabalin.
c. Lidocaine.
d. Diclofenac.
e. Clonidine.

72 A 76-year-old man is admitted with a short history of a dry mouth, diplopia and dysphagia. He develops a symmetrical descending weakness, initially affecting the trunk and proximal limb muscles, and spreading more peripherally. He has no sensory involvement. The most likely diagnosis is:

a. Tetanus.
b. Guillain-Barré syndrome.
c. Syringobulbia.
d. Botulism.
e. Myasthenia gravis.

73 A 56-year-old man is admitted with sepsis secondary to community-acquired pneumonia. He is treated with oxygen, intravenous antibiotics and repeated fluid challenges to a total volume of 4.5L (equivalent to 60ml/kg) of sodium chloride 0.9%. On reassessment, his pulse is 128 beats per minute, his blood pressure is 72/40mmHg (mean arterial pressure 54mmHg) and his respiratory rate is 28 breaths per minute. Oxygen saturation is 92% (94-99), breathing 50% oxygen. His central venous pressure is 12mmHg and his central venous oxygen saturation is 55%. His arterial blood gas shows a mild metabolic acidosis with a chloride of 112mEq/L, and a haemoglobin concentration of 83g/L. What is the next step in his cardiovascular optimisation?

a.   Transfuse packed red cells to a haematocrit of >30%.
b.   Dobutamine infusion.
c.   Colloid bolus.
d.   Switch to a balanced salt solution and continue fluid resuscitation.
e.   Norepinephrine infusion.

74 A trauma patient is admitted to the intensive care unit. He has sustained a traumatic brain injury with a small subdural haematoma and frontal contusions, several left-sided rib fractures and an open tibial fracture following a fall of 20 feet. The neurosurgical plan is for conservative management, intracranial pressure (ICP) monitoring and sedation for at least 48 hours. His ICP is currently 18mmHg. He underwent whole body CT imaging on admission, which has been reviewed by a consultant radiologist. The CT of his cervical spine has been reported as normal. He is currently in a hard collar. Which of the following is the most appropriate step in clinical management?

a. Change to Aspen collar.
b. Maintain in hard collar pending neurosurgical/spinal review.
c. Arrange magnetic resonance imaging to exclude ligamentous injury.
d. Maintain full in-line stabilisation until awake, fully conscious and able to clinically clear the cervical spine.
e. Discontinue immobilisation and nurse in midline.

75 A 41-year-old female presents with abdominal pain, nausea and vomiting, and diarrhoea. Examination shows her to be mildly jaundiced, in atrial fibrillation, and agitated, with bibasal crackles on chest auscultation and peripheral oedema. Observations include: heart rate 134 bpm, BP 76/45mmHg, respiratory rate 28, SaO_2 93% on air, temperature 39.6°C. She has mildly deranged liver function tests, a normal white cell count and C-reactive protein (CRP). A β-HCG test suggests she is pregnant. What is the most likely diagnosis?

a. Thyroid storm.
b. Decompensated alcoholic liver disease.
c. Sepsis.
d. Malaria.
e. Ectopic pregnancy.

76 A 43-year-old woman develops palpitations with chest pain on the coronary care unit. She receives sublingual glyceryl trinitrate (GTN) and intravenous diamorphine therapy with good effect. On examination, her blood pressure is 70/55mmHg, her respiratory rate is 30 breaths per minute and her oxygen saturation is 98% (94-99). A cardiac monitor shows a narrow-complex irregular tachycardia with a ventricular rate between 160 and 170 beats per minute. She has a wide-bore cannula *in situ* and high-flow oxygen is being administered. What is the most appropriate next step in management?

a.   Intravenous verapamil 5mg bolus.
b.   Carotid sinus massage.
c.   Intravenous amiodarone 300mg bolus over 5 minutes.
d.   Intravenous adenosine with cardiac monitoring (initial bolus 6mg).
e.   Synchronised DC cardioversion with sedation.

77 You are called for an opinion on a 52-year-old male in the emergency department who has been brought in by ambulance with new-onset dense right-sided hemiparesis and expressive dysphasia. He has no other cranial nerve signs on examination. His symptoms began 5 hours previously. There has been no loss of consciousness or seizure activity. His current GCS is E3 M5 V3. He has no other past medical history and is hypertensive at 179/95mmHg, but otherwise cardiovascularly stable.

a.   The patient has a partial anterior circulation infarct by the Bamford classification.

b. There is insufficient information provided to calculate a ROSIER score at this stage.

c. The patient should undergo emergent intubation and ventilation for 24 hours.

d. Should cranial imaging reveal no overt haemorrhage, he should receive intravenous thrombolysis in accordance with national guidelines.

e. In the presence of atrial fibrillation at presentation, immediate therapeutic anticoagulation should commence to reduce the risk of further embolic stroke.

78 A 49-year-old patient with an infective exacerbation of chronic obstructive pulmonary disease (COPD) presents to the emergency department with increased shortness of breath. Controlled oxygen, nebulised salbutamol and ipratropium, prednisolone and antibiotics are administered. After 1 hour of treatment he remains tachypnoeic, with a respiratory rate of 28, SpO_2 88% and GCS 15. An arterial blood gas (ABG) is performed which shows: pH 7.24, pCO_2 9.4kPa, pO_2 7.6kPa. He has not received any intravenous bronchodilators. The best treatment plan is:

a. Repeat nebulised salbutamol and ipratropium until clinical response.

b. Trial of non-invasive ventilation (NIV) in a critical care area.

c. Low-dose ketamine infusion.

d. Intravenous aminophylline loading.

e. Doxapram infusion.

79 A 19-year-old woman with a history of depression is brought to hospital by ambulance. Her father suspects she has taken an overdose of her medication. Her

Glasgow Coma Score is 11 (E3V4M4). Arterial blood gas analysis shows a glucose level of 6.7mmol/L and a mild metabolic acidosis. On arrival in the department she has a tonic-clonic seizure, which lasts for 2 minutes and then self-terminates. She remains post-ictal. ECG shows a broad-complex tachycardia with a heart rate of 120 beats per minute. What is the most appropriate immediate treatment?

a. Intravenous amiodarone.
b. DC cardioversion.
c. Intravenous sodium bicarbonate.
d. Intravenous lorazepam.
e. Intravenous esmolol infusion.

80 You are called to see a 77-year-old male patient with return of spontaneous circulation (ROSC) in the emergency department following an out-of-hospital cardiac arrest preceded by chest pain. Downtime was approximately 15 minutes during which he received bystander CPR immediately. His initial rhythm was pulseless ventricular tachycardia, which reverted with a single DC shock. He has no acute ECG changes and his blood pressure is 86/55mmHg unsupported. He was intubated by the paramedic team with evidence of soiling on laryngoscopy. His post-ROSC gas on 100% oxygen reveals a pH of 7.28, PO_2 of 22kPa, CO_2 of 6.3kPa, lactate of 3.2mmol/L, potassium of 3.4mmol/L and blood glucose of 8.3mmol/L. His GCS is 4. Temperature is recorded as 35.6°C via a tympanic thermometer. Cardiology review is awaited. What is the most appropriate next step in care?

a. Cool the patient to 32-34°C.
b. Load with aspirin, clopidogrel and fondaparinux.
c. Urgent bronchoscopy to assess for evidence of aspiration.
d. Arrange CT brain.
e. Titrate down the FiO_2.

81 An 81-year-old woman recently underwent cardiac surgery where temporary epicardial pacemaker wires were inserted. The pacemaker is set to DDD mode with a rate of 90 beats per minute (bpm). The nurse calls you as her observations are as follows: HR 35, BP 72/40mmHg, RR 16, SaO_2 96% on an FiO_2 0.5, GCS 13. Her ECG shows wide QRS complexes at a rate of 35 bpm; pacing spikes can be seen at a rate of 90 bpm. Your first action should be to:

a. Change the batteries in the pacemaker.
b. Increase the pacemaker prescribed rate.
c. Change to an alternate form of pacing.
d. Increase the voltage output from the pacemaker.
e. Decrease the pacemaker sensitivity.

82 A 57-year-old man presents with a 1-week history of increasing shortness of breath. He has a history of mild asthma, and chronic renal failure for which he received a renal transplant 5 years ago. His renal function has been stable apart from a recent episode of acute rejection which settled with treatment. He takes salbutamol and budesonide inhalers but these have not helped in recent days. He has minimal wheeze on chest auscultation, but has oxygen saturations of 89% on room air and a $PaCO_2$ of 3.7 on arterial blood gas analysis. Chest X-ray is slightly

hyper-inflated but lung fields are clear. Which investigation is likely to be diagnostic?

a. D-dimer level.
b. Atypical serology.
c. Bronchoalveolar lavage.
d. Ventilation/perfusion scan of the lungs.
e. Lung biopsy.

83 You are called to see a 35-year-old female on the surgical ward 24 hours after incision and drainage of a small thigh abscess. She is complaining of nausea and increasing pain and looks unwell. On examination she has a tachycardia of 140 bpm, temperature of 39.6°C and is hypotensive at 85/30mmHg. She is sweaty and agitated. She has an intravenous line *in situ* and is currently receiving normal saline at 100ml/hr and paracetamol intravenously. On assessment, she is confused but has a clear chest, normal heart sounds, soft abdomen and no obvious external wounds. The first priority should be:

a. Intravenous dantrolene.
b. Administer β-lactam and clindamycin antibiotics.
c. Urgent CT imaging of the thigh.
d. Administer intravenous immunoglobulin.
e. Arrange urgent general surgical review.

84 A 69-year-old patient is admitted to the surgical ward with abdominal pain. He has a pH of 7.15, lactate of 6mmol/L and has had a period of hypotension. He undergoes laparotomy where a segment of ischaemic small bowel is resected and an end-to-end anastomosis is performed. Following admission (ventilated) to the intensive care unit, his metabolic acidosis and raised lactate resolve overnight following fluid resuscitation with 4L of crystalloid. Twenty-four hours after admission his urine output drops to <0.5ml/kg/hr and his urea and creatinine start to rise. He develops an ileus and his nasogastric tube is put on free drainage. His serum potassium is 5.2mmol/L, pH 7.23. Intra-abdominal pressure is 27mmHg. Haemodynamic monitoring shows: blood pressure 123/76mmHg, cardiac index 4.5L/min/m^2, systemic vascular resistance index 2100 dyne/sec/cm^5/m^2, stroke volume variation 8%. Which of the options below is the most appropriate course of action to treat the underlying cause of this patient's deterioration?

a. Renal replacement therapy.
b. Fluid bolus.
c. Dopamine infusion.
d. Return to theatre for laparostomy.
e. Increase sedation and neuromuscular blockade.

85 A 46-year-old man's house is on fire and he is brought into the emergency department with partial-thickness skin burns. The ICU physician is asked to assess him in the emergency department resuscitation room. Fluid has been prescribed according to the Parkland formula. Which of the following is the best endpoint for initial crystalloid titration?

a. Central venous pressure of 8-12mmHg.
b. Clinical assessment of hydration.
c. Mean arterial pressure.
d. Heart rate.
e. Urine output.

86 You are asked to admit a 48-year-old female patient with acute-on-chronic liver disease and grade III encephalopathy. She has been admitted under the medical team with acute kidney injury and deteriorating liver function tests. There is no clear precipitant for decompensation on history from the family. They also state that she continues to drink heavily. On review, she has normal oxygen saturations on FiO_2 of 0.4 with a PO_2 of 10kPa. She is hypotensive at 76/40mmHg and tachycardic at 110 bpm. A catheter is *in situ* and she has passed 20ml of urine over the last 8 hours. Her bilirubin today is 230μmol/L and alanine transaminase is 56μmol/L. Serum creatinine is 478μmol/L. Which of the following prognostic systems is likely to be the best predictor of outcome in this patient?

a. Modified End-stage Liver Disease (MELD) score.
b. Child-Pugh score.
c. APACHE II score.
d. Sequential Organ Failure Assessment (SOFA) score.
e. Glasgow Alcohol Score.

87 A 71-year-old man is admitted to the intensive care unit with severe sepsis secondary to community-acquired pneumonia. He develops multi-organ failure. Following ventilation for 16 days, attempts to wean from ventilation are unsuccessful. Examination shows diffuse weakness and hyporeflexia. Electrophysiological investigations show normal conduction velocities, a decrease in compound muscle action potential (CMAP) amplitude and a normal sensory nerve action potential (SNAP) amplitude with a 5% decrement of CMAP amplitude on repetitive nerve stimulation and no increment response on exercise of the muscles. His CSF protein levels are normal. What is the most likely cause for this patient's weakness?

a. Critical illness polyneuropathy.
b. Critical illness myopathy.
c. Guillain-Barré syndrome.
d. Myasthenia gravis.
e. Lambert-Eaton syndrome.

88 A man is admitted with a severe chest infection. He consents to a HIV test. Which of the following is not an AIDS-defining illness?

a. Mycobacteria tuberculosis.
b. Kaposi's sarcoma.
c. Cerebral lymphoma.
d. *Cytomegalovirus* (CMV) retinitis.
e. Oral candidiasis.

89 You are asked to see a 35-year-old female patient, brought to the emergency department following a house fire. She was retrieved from the bedroom unconscious with no evidence of injury. On arrival, she had a GCS of 4 with sluggish dilated pupils and laboured breathing and so underwent immediate uncomplicated endotracheal intubation via rapid sequence induction. On assessment, she has an SpO$_2$ of 99% on FiO$_2$ 1.0 and some scattered crepitations throughout the chest but no wheeze. She is hypotensive at 82/45mmHg via non-invasive blood pressure measurement and tachycardic at 105 bpm. There is no evidence of thoracoabdominal, pelvic or long bone trauma and no external burns on secondary survey. She has two intravenous lines and crystalloid running at 250ml/hr, alongside sedation.

Her post-intubation arterial blood gas comes back with the following values: pH 7.1, PO_2 54.3kPa, PCO_2 4.5kPa, HCO_3^- 15mmol/L, base excess -8mmol/L, lactate 14mmol/L, carboxyhaemoglobin 15%. Which of the following management options is likely to be of most benefit?

a. Immediate transfer for whole body CT.
b. IV fluid bolus.
c. Titrate the oxygen to a PO_2 of 8-10kPa.
d. Transfer for hyperbaric oxygen therapy.
e. Administration of hydroxocobalamin.

90 A 78-year-old female is admitted to the high dependency unit following elective thyroidectomy. She has multiple comorbidities and very limited exercise capacity. She does well and that evening she is sitting out of bed having dinner when she develops a rapidly expanding haematoma over the anterior aspect of her neck and complains of difficulty breathing. On examination she has a heart rate of 114 bpm, blood pressure of 103/68mmHg, a capillary refill time of 3 seconds, SaO_2 91% on 30% oxygen and stridor can be heard. Releasing the sutures from her neck wound makes no difference to her signs and symptoms. She is extremely agitated and trying to climb out of bed. What is the most appropriate method of securing her airway?

a. Administering propofol and atracurium, then using direct laryngoscopy for intubation with an endotracheal tube.
b. Rapid sequence induction.
c. Awake tracheostomy under local anaesthetic.
d. Gas induction.
e. Awake fibreoptic intubation.

Paper 3
Answers

1 F, F, F, F, F

Non-invasive ventilation (NIV) has been the subject of many randomised controlled trials in various patient groups. The strongest evidence for its use is in patients with Type II respiratory failure secondary to exacerbation of chronic obstructive pulmonary disease (COPD) where there is a large mortality benefit compared with usual medical care. Its role in asthma is not well established, and is not recommended in consensus guidelines for patients with a worsening respiratory acidosis who should be intubated. There is no good quality evidence to suggest a benefit in pneumonia, especially where there is a high secretion burden, although NIV may have a role in selected patients who would not be for escalation to mechanical ventilation. While planned extubation directly onto NIV is a reasonable weaning strategy, the use of NIV as a rescue therapy in cases of failed intubation has been shown not to be effective. NIV is not contraindicated in thoracic wall deformities and may be a valuable strategy to avoid the need for intubation in selected patients.

1. Ram FS, Picot J, Lightowler J, et al. Non-invasive positive pressure ventilation for treatment of respiratory failure due to exacerbations of chronic obstructive pulmonary disease. Cochrane Database Syst Rev 2004; 1: CD004104.
2. British Thoracic Society & Scottish Intercollegiate Guidelines Network. British guideline on the management of asthma, 2014. http://www.sign.ac.uk/pdf/QRG141.pdf (accessed 7th January 2015).
3. Esteban A, Frutos-Vivar F, Ferguson ND, et al. Noninvasive positive-pressure ventilation for respiratory failure after extubation. New Engl J Med 2004; 350: 2542-60.

2   F, F, F, F, F

The National Institute for Health and Care Excellence (NICE) guidance suggests <0.5 x 10^9/L as the cut-off for neutropaenia, unless the count is <1 x 10^9/L and falling. Aminoglycosides are contraindicated as empirical therapy unless specific microbiological recommendations exist. Indwelling catheters can be left *in situ* in the first instance, but should be cultured to guide specific therapy. Glycopeptide antibiotics are not recommended for those patients with central vascular access devices unless specific patient or local microbiological recommendations exist.

Empirical G-CSF is not recommended, as per NICE guidance. However, some cancer networks will recommend early G-CSF for patients with high-risk conditions and neutropenic sepsis, including multi-organ failure, hypotension and age >65. Secondary prophylaxis can also be considered following an episode of febrile neutropenia, to prevent further treatment delays based on the failure of neutrophil count to recover.

1.   Phillips R, Hancock B, Graham J, *et al. Prevention and management of neutropenic sepsis in patients with cancer: summary of NICE guidance. Br Med J* 2013; 345: e5368.

3   F, T, T, F, F

The anterior triangle of the neck is bounded posteriorly by the medial border of the sternocleidomastoid and anteriorly by the midline. The carotid sheath passes through the anterior triangle and contains the common, internal and part of the external carotid arteries, the internal jugular vein and parts of the glossopharyngeal, vagus and accessory nerves. The internal carotid artery can be palpated at the inferior border of the mandible. For central venous access, the skin is punctured at the apex of the two heads of the sternocleidomastoid; by definition this is in the posterior triangle of the neck.

1.   Gosling JA, Harris PF, Humpherson JR, *et al. Human Anatomy Color Atlas and Text*, 3rd ed. London, UK: Mosby-Wolfe, 1996.

4 F, F, T, T, T

Hypercalcaemia has numerous causes. The commonest are primary hyperparathyroidism (due to solitary adenoma, hyperplasia or as part of MEN syndromes I and IIa) and malignancy. Elevated calcium levels in malignancy may be due to the production of parathyroid hormone-related protein (PTHrP) or bony metastasis. Other rarer causes include vitamin D-mediated (including sarcoidosis and excessive ingestion) and drug causes such as thiazide diuretics, lithium, theophyllines, thyroxine and vitamin D. Immobilisation is a rarer cause of hypercalcaemia and is secondary to increased bone resorption. Hyperthyroidism is a recognised cause of hypercalcaemia, although less common than hyperparathyroidism. The mechanism is not entirely clear, but may involve up-regulation of osteoclast activity.

1.   Ramrakah P, Moore K. Endocrine emergencies. *Oxford Handbook of Acute Medicine*, 3rd ed. Oxford, UK: Oxford University Press, 2010.

5 T, F, F, F, F

Low, high and variable sugar control carry a clear risk to the critical care patient. Indeed, the risk of mortality is suggested to increase with the severity and duration of dysglycaemia in a dose-dependent fashion. A sustained approach to therapy is needed.

The paradigm shift in approach to glycaemic control in critical care is an excellent example of medical reversal within the last 20 years. With the original Leuven trials, tight glycaemic control was widely adopted on the supposition from single-centre trial evidence that mortality would decrease. This was later contradicted by both the VISEP (Efficacy of Volume Substitution and Insulin Therapy in Severe Sepsis) and NICE-SUGAR (Normoglycemia in Intensive Care Evaluation and Surviving Using Glucose Algorithm Regulation) studies, which provided level I evidence to show no benefit from tight glycaemic control and also suggested an increased rate of complications secondary to hypoglycaemic episodes. A post-hoc analysis of NICE-SUGAR has recently confirmed the risk of hypoglycaemia with tight control to be ten times that of conventional therapy.

Standard targets for conventional glycaemic control are now <10mmol/L, based on the NICE-SUGAR protocol.

1.   Badawi O, Waite MD, Fuhrman SA, Zuckerman IH. Association between intensive care unit-acquired dysglycaemia and in-hospital mortality. *Crit Care Med* 2012; 40(12): 3180-8.
2.   Van den Berghe G, Wouters P, Weekers F, *et al*. Intensive insulin therapy in critically ill patients. *New Engl J Med* 2001; 345(19): 1359-67.
3.   Van den Berghe G, Wilmer A, Hermans G, *et al*. Intensive insulin therapy in the medical ICU. *New Engl J Med* 2006; 354(5): 449-61.
4.   Brunkhorst FM, Engel C, Bloos F, *et al*. Intensive insulin therapy and pentastarch resuscitation in severe sepsis. *New Engl J Med* 2008; 358(2): 125-39.
5.   NICE-SUGAR study investigators. Intensive versus conventional glucose control in critically ill patients. *New Engl J Med* 2009; 360(13): 1283-97.
6.   NICE-SUGAR study investigators. Hypoglycaemia and risk of death in critically ill patients. *New Engl J Med* 2012; 367(12): 1108-18.

6   T, T, F, T, F

Drug dosages are equivalent when administered via the intravenous and intraosseous routes. The humerus and tibia have equal flow rates for fluids. Tracheal administration leads to variable plasma concentrations of drugs and with the advent of newer devices making IO access easier, tracheal drug administration is no longer recommended.

1.   Resuscitation Council (UK). Resuscitation guidelines 2010. London, UK: Resuscitation Council (UK). http://www.resus.org.uk/pages/guide.htm (accessed 25th February 2015).

7   T, T, T, F, F

The laryngeal mask airway (LMA) is a supraglottic airway device developed by British anaesthetist Dr. Archie Brain. It has been in use since 1988. The LMA is shaped like a large endotracheal tube on the proximal end that connects to an elliptical mask on the distal end. It is designed to sit in the patient's hypopharynx and cover the supraglottic structures, thereby allowing relative isolation of the trachea.

The LMA is a good airway device in many settings, because it is easy to use even for the inexperienced provider. Its use results in less gastric distension than with bag-valve-mask ventilation, which reduces but does not eliminate the risk of aspiration. This may be particularly pertinent in patients who have not fasted before being ventilated. It can be safely used for longer procedures including those requiring positive pressure ventilation.

After failed intubation due to difficult laryngoscopy, the LMA can be used as a rescue device. In the case of the patient who cannot be intubated but can be ventilated, the LMA is a good alternative to continued bag-valve-mask ventilation because it is easier to maintain over time and it has been shown to decrease, though not eliminate, aspiration risk.

The 2005 American Heart Association guidelines indicate the LMA as an acceptable alternative to intubation for airway management in the cardiac arrest patient (Class IIa). This may be particularly useful in the pre-hospital setting, where emergency medical technicians typically have less experience with intubation and lower success rates.

Absolute contraindications (in all settings, including emergent):

- Cannot open mouth.
- Complete upper airway obstruction.

Relative contraindications:

- Increased risk of aspiration:
    - prolonged bag-valve-mask ventilation;
    - morbid obesity;
    - second or third trimester pregnancy;
    - patients who have not fasted before ventilation;
    - upper gastrointestinal bleed.
- Suspected or known abnormalities in supraglottic anatomy.
- Need for high airway pressures.

Induction of anaesthesia or heavy sedation with any of the common induction agents facilitate insertion. Propofol is especially suitable as it suppresses laryngeal reflexes facilitating placement of the device. Neuromuscular blockade is not required.

1. Bosson N, Byrd Jr RP. Laryngeal mask airway. http//www.emedicine.medscape.com/article/82527-overview (accessed 25th February 2015).

8   T, F, F, F, F

There has been much focus on rescue therapies for severe hypoxaemia in acute respiratory distress syndrome (ARDS) over the last 20 years. An emerging evidence base is developing and continues to guide best practice.

Early neuromuscular blockade to support invasive ventilation and decrease metabolic requirement has recently been shown to reduce mortality and the duration of mechanical ventilation in patients with severe ARDS. Therapeutic hypothermia has no evidence base to support its use in this condition. High-frequency oscillatory ventilation (HFOV) has recently been the subject of two large randomised controlled trials (RCTs) and found to offer no benefit to conventional mechanical ventilation.

Airway pressure release ventilation (APRV) and inhaled nitric oxide have both been purported as rescue measures for severe disease. However, the current evidence has not demonstrated any evidence of benefit and their role in management remains limited.

1. Papazian L, Forel JM, Gacouin A, *et al*. Neuromuscular blockers in early acute respiratory distress syndrome. *N Engl J Med* 2010; 363: 1107-16.
2. Young D, Lamb SE, Shah S, *et al*. High frequency oscillatory ventilation for the acute respiratory distress syndrome. *N Engl J Med* 2013; 368: 806-13.
3. Ferguson ND, Cook DJ, Guyatt GH, *et al*. High frequency oscillation in early acute respiratory distress syndrome. *N Engl J Med* 2013; 368: 795-805.
4. Adhikari NK, Dellinger RP, Lundin S, *et al*. Inhaled nitric oxide does not reduce mortality in patients with acute respiratory distress syndrome regardless of severity: systematic review and meta-analysis. *Crit Care Med* 2014; 42(2): 404-12.

9   F, T, F, F, T

Immediately life-threatening injuries which should be identified and managed during the primary survey are: tension pneumothorax, open pneumothorax, flail chest, massive haemothorax and cardiac tamponade. Whilst other injuries are also potentially lethal they should be identified and managed during the secondary survey.

1.   American College of Surgeons Committee on Trauma. *Advanced Trauma Life Support for Doctors, ATLS, Student Course Manual*, 8th ed. Chicago, USA: American College of Surgeons, 2008.

10   T, F, T, T, F

The thromboelastogram (TEG®) provides information of global haemostatic function rather than the measurements of prothrombin time (PT) and activated partial thromboplastin time (aPTT). It is a graphical representation of the mechanics of clot formation assessed by the degree of traction on a pin suspended in a spinning cup of blood. A normal TEG® is shown in Figure 3.1. Normal values are shown in Table 3.1.

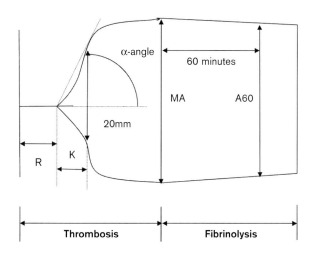

Figure 3.1. A normal TEG®.

Table 3.1. Normal values of a TEG®.

	Value	Physiological process	Blood component
R-time (reaction)	8-12 minutes	Initial fibrin formation rate	Plasma clotting factors and inhibitor activity
K-time (clot formation)	2-4 minutes (curve amplitude 20mm)	Fibrin accumulation and cross-linkage	Fibrinogen, platelets and intrinsic clotting factors
α (slope from R to K) angle	60-70°	Speed of solid clot formation	Thrombocytopaenia and hypofibrinogenaemia decrease angle
MA (maximum amplitude)	60-70mm	Absolute strength of fibrin clot	Platelet number, function and fibrin interaction
LY30 (% lysis of clot 30 minutes after maximum amplitude)	<7.5%	Loss of clot integrity due to lysis. Reflects fibrinolysis.	
A60 (amplitude 60 minutes after MA)	MA — 5mm	Clot retraction lysis	

Various algorithms exist to guide blood product replacement in cases with an abnormal TEG®. In general, a prolonged R-time may indicate requirement for fresh frozen plasma, a reduced MA suggests platelets are required and a low MA 60 minutes later may indicate hyperfibrinolysis consistent with disseminated intravascular coagulation. (NB: the normal values above are based on a kaolin-activated blood sample; a slightly different reference range exists for whole blood.)

1.   Curry A, Pierce J. Conventional and near-patient tests of coagulation. *Contin Educ Anaesth Crit Care Pain* 2007; 7: 45-50.

11   F, T, F, F, F

Odds and risk are differentiated by the denominator, which is the proportion without the condition of interest for the former and the total population of interest for the latter. The number needed to treat (NNT) is calculated using 1/absolute risk reduction (ARR), when ARR is the control event rate minus the experimental event rate. Type I error refers to the chance of a false-positive result within a trial and Type II the possibility of a false-negative result. The latter commonly arises due to limitations in sample size, whereas the former can occur due to sources of bias, such as problems with allocation concealment, randomisation, selection and observer bias.

A funnel plot assesses the existence of publication bias within systematic reviews. Study results are charted with the assumption that larger trials will be plotted near the average with smaller trials dotted either side, thus forming a funnel-shape distribution. Heterogeneity is usually assessed using the I2 value.

Laboratory or experimental hypothesis testing studies look to assess efficacy (proof of concept). Large clinical trials look for evidence of effectiveness (proof of effect within the population of interest). An intention to treat analysis incorporates all those randomised to receive the treatment within the study group results, rather than just those who actually received/completed the medication course. This can highlight difficulties in therapeutics as a result of side effects, cost, or patient choice and, as such, is a useful tool to assess the potential for a new medication to be effective within a 'real world' cohort.

1.   Goodacre S. Critical appraisal for emergency medicine 3: evaluation of a therapy. *Emerg Med J* 2008; 25: 590-2.

12   F, F, F, F, F

There are several systems used to assess trauma. They assess physiological and anatomical data to provide triage tools and information for outcome databases. The Abbreviated Injury Scale (AIS) grades an injury from 1 — minor, to 6 — unsurvivable. The intervals between the scores are not consistent, but the higher the score the worse the injury. The Injury Severity Score is an anatomical scoring system that provides a score for patients with multiple injuries. Each injury is assigned an AIS score and assigned to one of 6 body regions: head, face, chest, abdomen, extremities and external. The score for the highest AIS in each region is used. The three highest scoring regions are identified, their scores are squared and then summed. Values range from 0-75. Any injury assigned an AIS of 6 automatically denotes an ISS of 75. The Revised Trauma Score (RTS) is a physiological scoring system. Developed from a North American trauma database using regression analysis, it grades the parameters of respiratory rate, systolic blood pressure and Glasgow Coma Scale score. It delivers a score between 0 and 12 and tends to be used as a triage tool. TRISS determines the probability of survival of a patient and is calculated using a mathematical formula which incorporates the ISS, RTS, an age index and mechanism of injury (blunt or penetrating trauma).

1.   Lecky F, Woodford M, Edwards A, *et al*. Trauma scoring systems and databases. *Br J Anaesth* 2014; 113(2): 286-94.
2.   Trauma Score - Injury Severity Score: TRISS. http://www.trauma.org/archive/scores/triss.html (accessed 15th August 2014).

13   F, T, T, F, T

Pleural fluid is normally yellow in appearance. It can be haemorrhagic in trauma, pulmonary infarction and malignancies. Turbid or purulent fluid suggests a parapneumonic effusion or empyema. A pleural protein level of <30g/L is seen in transudative pleural effusions, whereas a pleural fluid protein level of >30g/L suggests an exudative effusion. Care should be taken in interpreting this result if the serum total protein is abnormal.

Causes of transudative pleural effusions include heart failure, protein-losing enteropathy, nephrotic syndrome, hypothyroidism and fluid overload. Causes of exudative pleural effusions include parapneumonic effusions, empyema, oesophageal rupture, subphrenic abscess, pancreatitis, malignancy and pulmonary embolism.

The pleural fluid protein should be measured to differentiate between a transudative and exudative pleural effusion. This will usually suffice if the patient's serum protein is normal and pleural protein is less than 25g/L or more than 35g/L. If not, Light's criteria should be used. Unfortunately, the protein level often lies very close to the 30g/L cut-off point, making clear differentiation difficult. In these cases, measurement of serum and pleural fluid lactate dehydrogenase (LDH) and total protein levels will allow the use of Light's criteria to distinguish between these two more accurately.

Light's criteria

The pleural fluid is an exudate if one or more of the following criteria are met:

- Pleural fluid protein divided by serum protein >0.5.
- Pleural fluid LDH divided by serum LDH >0.6.
- Pleural fluid LDH more than two thirds the upper limits of normal serum LDH.

Low glucose levels in pleural effusions occur in bacterial infections, rheumatoid arthritis, malignancy and systemic lupus erythematosus (SLE).

1. Maskell NA, Butland RJA, on behalf of the British Thoracic Society Pleural Disease Group, a subgroup of the British Thoracic Society Standards of Care Committee. BTS guidelines for the investigation of a unilateral pleural effusion in adults. *Thorax* 2003; 58: ii8-17.
2. Bersten AD, Soni N. *Oh's Intensive Care Manual*, 6th ed. Philadelphia, USA: Butterworth Heinemann, Elsevier, 2009.

14   F, T, T, T, F

The recommended energy for DC cardioversion is 4J/kg at present. The formula to estimate weight has been the subject of much debate and recently changed within the recent Advanced Paediatric Life Support (APLS) guidelines from the standard 2 x (age + 4) to that proposed by Luscombe and Owens. The latter formula is segregated by age as below:

- Infant — (0.5 x age in months)+4.
- 1-5 years — (2 x age in years)+8.
- 6-12 years — (3 x age in years)+7.

Several studies support the change, including the recent results of the CORKSCREW (CORK Study of Children's Realistic Estimation of Weight) project, amongst others. There is still debate regarding the merits for formula estimation against maternal estimate or rapid weight assessment on admission.

Amiodarone for VT is dosed at 5mg/kg and empirical ceftriaxone for suspected meningococcus at 80mg/kg.

The suggested APLS formula for the internal diameter of a suitable endotracheal tube is currently Cole's formula — (age/4)+4 — as reported in 1957 originally. There is current debate regarding the suitability of cuffed tube placement in all paediatric patients and the use of a modified Cole's formula to predict internal diameter.

1. Luscombe M, Owens B. Weight estimation in resuscitation: is the current formula still valid? *Arch Dis Child* 2007; 92(5): 412-5.
2. Skrobo D, Kelleher G. CORKSCREW 2013 - the CORK Study of Children's Realistic Estimation of Weight. *Emerg Med J* 2015; 32(1): 32-5.
3. http://www.stemlynsblog.org/apls-estimation-formulas-do-not-safely-predict-weight-in-uk-children (accessed 26th February 2015).
4. Cole F. Pediatric formulas for the anaesthesiologist. *AMA J Dis Child* 1957; 94: 672-3.
5. Clements RS, Steel AG, Bates AT, Mackenzie R. Cuffed endotracheal tube use in paediatric prehospital intubation: challenging the doctrine? *Emerg Med J* 2007; 24(1): 57-8.

15 F, T, F, F, F

Effective hand washing involves three stages: preparation (wetting hands and applying soap), washing (rubbing hands together vigorously for 10-15 seconds) and drying (using paper towels). Alcohol-based hand rub is not effective against all micro-organisms, including some viruses (such as Norovirus) and spore-forming micro-organisms (such as *Clostridium difficile*). After a procedure, gloves, then apron, then eye protection and then mask/respirator should be removed, in that order, to minimise the risk of cross/self-contamination. Urinary tract infection is the most common infection acquired as a result of healthcare. Catheters predispose to infection because micro-organisms are able to bypass natural host mechanisms and gain entry to the bladder. The bladder is normally sterile, but after a few days of catheterisation, micro-organisms may be isolated from the urine — 'bacteriuria'. After 2-10 days, approximately 30% of catheterised patients will develop bacteriuria. Dressings on CVCs should be changed after 7 days, or earlier if visibly contaminated.

1. Loveday HP, Wilson JA, Pratt RJ, *et al*. epic3: National evidence-based guidelines for preventing healthcare-associated infections in NHS hospitals in England. *J Hosp Infect* 2014; 86: S1-70.

16   F, T, F, F, F

Necrotising fasciitis (NF) is a progressive overwhelming bacterial infection of subcutaneous tissue. It spreads rapidly and therefore early diagnosis and intervention are essential. Delays in definitive treatment (surgical debridement) increase tissue loss, and mortality rate.

Clinically, pain typically precedes skin changes by 24-48 hours and normal-looking skin is quite commonly seen early in the disease process. Significant muscle involvement is frequently not present and is not a diagnostic feature. Differential diagnosis may include muscular pain and cellulitis but a high index of suspicion for NF must be maintained given the high mortality rate. The Laboratory Risk Indicator for Necrotising Fasciitis (LRINEC) scoring system was designed to distinguish NF from other soft tissue infections. This classifies NF into four subtypes:

* Type 1 — the most common. Polymicrobial including a combination of Gram-positive cocci, Gram-negative rods, and anaerobes.
* Type 2 — caused by the group A *Streptococcus* (*Streptococcus pyogenes*) either alone or in association with *Staphylococcus aureus*, the only type associated with toxic shock syndrome and staphylococcal infections.

- Type 3 — rare in occurrence, caused by Gram-negative bacteria most commonly *Vibrio* species.
- Type 4 — fungal (usually *Candida spp*), rare and seen in immunocompromised patients, and those with traumatic burns and wounds.

1. Davoudian P, Flint NJ. Necrotising fasciitis. *Contin Educ Anaesth Crit Care Pain* 2012; 12(5): 245-50.

17 T, F, T, F, F

Clinical clearance of the cervical spine is best attempted using the Canadian C Spine Decision Rule (CCR), which was designed following a logistic regression analysis of >8000 patients and has proven superior to other tools, such as the NEXUS criteria. This tool mandates radiography in all patients >65, with peripheral paraesthesiae or a dangerous mechanism of injury. As such, these patient groups cannot be clinically cleared, and must undergo radiological clearance in the context of suspected injury.

Recent NICE head injury guidance has adjusted recommendations on cervical spine imaging, to suggest that the majority of trauma patients should undergo CT assessment rather than three plain view X-rays, based on the limited sensitivity of the latter. Rates of occult injury on MR imaging in the obtunded trauma patient with a negative CT cervical spine have been reported as anywhere between 1-5%, but the number of injuries that need subsequent treatment is negligible.

Three-point immobilisation has a very limited evidence base and many pre-hospital services are beginning to discontinue its practice, in light of the discomfort, harm and cost. No immobilisation strategy has shown any benefit in the case of soft tissue neck injury following trauma.

1. Stiell IG, Clement CM, McKnight RD, *et al.* The Canadian C-Spine Rule versus the NEXUS low-risk criteria in patients with trauma. *New Engl J Med* 2003; 349: 2510-8.
2. The National Institute for Health and Care Excellence. Triage, assessment, investigation and early management of head injury in children, young people and adults. NICE

clinical guideline 176. London, UK: NICE, 2014. www.nice.org.uk (accessed 25th February 2015).

3. Hogan GJ, Mirvis SE, Shanmuganathan K, Scalea TM. Exclusion of unstable cervical spine injury in obtunded patients with blunt trauma: is MR imaging needed when multi-detector row CT findings are normal? *Radiology* 2005; 237(1): 106-13.

4. Como JJ, Thompson MA, Anderson JS, *et al.* Is magnetic resonance imaging essential in clearing the cervical spine in obtunded patients with blunt trauma? *J Trauma* 2007; 63(3): 544-9.

18 F, T, T, F, T

Table 3.2. Calculation of predictive values for a diagnostic test.

	Has the disease	Does not have the disease	
Test result positive	a True positive	b False positive	Positive predictive value a/a+b
Test result negative	c False negative	d True negative	Negative predictive value c/d+c
	Sensitivity a/a+c	Specificity d/d+b	

Sensitivity of a clinical test refers to the ability of the test to correctly identify those patients with the disease. Specificity of a clinical test refers to the ability of the test to correctly identify those patients without the disease. Unlike sensitivity and specificity, the positive predictive value (PPV) and the negative predictive value (NPV) are dependent on the population being tested and are influenced by the prevalence of the disease. Screening for an illness in the general population using a certain test may have a low PPV due to the high number of false positives. If the test is performed in a population who are exhibiting signs of the disease, the PPV of the test increases. Receiver operator curves take into account the cut-off points for a particular test. If the cut-off point is raised, there are fewer false positives but more false negatives — the test is highly specific but not very sensitive. If the cut-off point is low, there are fewer false negatives but more false positives — the test is highly sensitive but not very specific. Receiver operator curves are a plot (1-specificity) of a test on the x-axis against the sensitivity on the y-axis for all possible cut-off points. The area under the curve represents the overall accuracy of a test, with a value approaching 1.0 indicating a high sensitivity and specificity. The line of zero discrimination has an area under the curve of 0.5 and is seen as a straight line on the graph.

1.   Lalkhen AG, McClusky AM. Clinical tests: sensitivity and specificity. *Contin Educ Anaesth Crit Care Pain* 2008; 8(6): 221-3.

19   T, F, F, F, T

Hypertrophic cardiomyopathy (HCM) is a commonly inherited cardiac disorder and common cause of death in young athletes with an annual mortality of 1-2%. It is caused by genetic mutations of sarcomeric proteins such as the β-myosin heavy chain and troponin. It is characterised by left ventricular hypertrophy in the absence of hypertension or aortic stenosis, and this is the commonest echocardiographic feature. The hypertrophy is usually asymmetrical, particularly affecting the anterior septal wall of the left ventricle. The most common cause of left ventricular outflow tract (LVOT) obstruction in HCM is systolic anterior motion of the mitral valve (SAM). However, nearly 70% of cases do not have LVOT obstruction, explaining the change of name from hypertrophic obstructive cardiomyopathy (HOCM) to HCM. β-blockade and the avoidance of hypovolaemia are the mainstays of treatment in preventing SAM.

Symptoms may include: exertional syncope or pre-syncope worsening chest pain, heart failure, palpitations due to arrhythmias such as supraventricular or ventricular tachyarrhythmias explaining the cause of sudden death.

There is an association between HCM and Wolff-Parkinson-White syndrome with at least one gene mutation occurring in both conditions. Adenosine monophosphate-activated protein kinase (AMPK) gene mutations cause HCM with Wolff-Parkinson-White syndrome and conduction disease.

1.   Maron BJ. Hypertrophic cardiomyopathy. *Lancet* 1997; 350(9071): 127-33.
2.   Kelly BS, Mattu A, Brady WJ. Hypertrophic cardiomyopathy: electrocardiographic manifestations and other important considerations for the emergency physician. *Am J Emerg Med* 2007; 25(1): 72-9.

20   F, T, F, F, F

A penetrating neck injury is defined as one that penetrates the underlying platysma muscle and can be segregated into a zone 1, 2 or 3 injury depending on anatomical location. Zone 1 is bordered by the thoracic inlet caudally and the cricoid cartilage cephalad; zone 2 extends from the cricoid cartilage to the angle of the mandible, and zone 3 extends from the angle of the mandible to the base of the skull. Previously, zone 2 injuries mandated surgical exploration. However, despite the potentially serious consequences of this injury pattern, mandatory exploration has been shown to result in a high proportion of 'negative' surgery. As such, recent guidelines have focused on early imaging, clinical assessment and selective operative management, with a level I recommendation.

CT imaging is reported to be highly sensitive for the detection of clinically significant vascular injuries in this patient cohort, with CT angiography having essentially replaced contrast arteriography as the investigation of choice. This modality is less sensitive for aerodigestive tract injury when performed early; if the patient deteriorates, oesophagoscopy or bronchoscopy should therefore be considered even in the presence of a negative CT. A systematic review has provided evidence regarding the limitations of cervical spine immobilisation via hard collar in this cohort and recommends use only with neurological deficit.

Dysphonia is considered as a 'soft' clinical sign along with oropharyngeal blood, haemoptysis and several others. 'Hard' signs (often used as a triage tool to mandate operative exploration) include subcutaneous emphysema/ bubbling air through the wound, airway compromise, expanding or pulsatile haematoma, active bleeding, neurological deficit or haematemesis.

1. Tisherman SA, Bokhari F, Collier B, *et al*. Clinical practice guideline: penetrating zone 2 neck trauma. *J Trauma* 2008; 64: 1392-405.
2. Inaba K, Branco BC, Menaker J, *et al*. Evaluation of multidetector computed tomography for penetrating neck injury: a prospective multicentre study. *J Trauma Acute Care Surg* 2012; 72(3): 576-83.
3. Kruger C, Lecky F. Is cervical spine protection always necessary following penetrating neck injury? *Emerg Med J* 2009; 26: 883-7.
4. Sperry JL, Moore EE, Coimbra R, *et al*. Western trauma association critical decisions in trauma: penetrating neck trauma. *J Trauma Acute Care Surg* 2013; 75(6): 936-40.

21   T, T, T, F, F

Right ventricular hypertrophy can be due to pulmonary hypertension, mitral stenosis, pulmonary embolism, chronic lung disease, congenital heart disease and arrhythmogenic right ventricular cardiomyopathy. Diagnostic ECG criteria for right ventricular hypertrophy include:

*   QRS duration <120ms.
*   Right axis deviation of +110° or more.
*   Dominant R-wave in V1 (>7mm tall or R/S ratio >1).
*   Dominant S-wave in V5 or V6 (>7mm tall or R/S ratio <1).

Supporting criteria for right ventricular hypertrophy include:

*   Right atrial enlargement (P pulmonale).
*   Right ventricular strain pattern = ST depression/T-wave inversion in the right precordial (V1-4) and inferior (II, III, aVF) leads.
*   S1, S2, S3 pattern = far right axis deviation with dominant S-waves in leads I, II and III.
*   Deep S-waves in the lateral leads (I, aVL, V5-6).

Bifid P waves are a sign of left atrial enlargement, which would support a diagnosis of left ventricular hypertrophy. ST depression/T-wave inversion in leads looking at the left side of the heart (V4-6) is a sign of left ventricular hypertrophy.

1. Harrigan RA, Jones K. Conditions affecting the right side of the heart. *Br Med J* 2002; 324(7347): 1201-4.

22   F, F, F, T, T

Status epilepticus is defined as continuous seizure activity of at least 30 minutes duration or intermittent seizure activity of at least 30 minutes duration during which consciousness is not regained. Management consists of attention to Airway, Breathing and Circulation and pharmacological intervention. First-line would be intravenous lorazepam, second-line phenytoin and, third-line, induction of anaesthesia with propofol, thiopentone or midazolam. Neuromuscular blocking drugs will be required to secure the airway but will not terminate seizure activity. Sodium valproate is a reasonable choice but not advocated in the 2012 NICE guidelines.

1. The National Institute for Health and Care Excellence. The epilepsies: the diagnosis and management of the epilepsies in adults and children in primary and secondary care: Appendix F. NICE clinical guideline 137. London, UK: NICE, 2012. www.nice.org.uk (accessed 25th February 2015).

23   T, F, T, F, F

Prognostication post-cardiac arrest syndrome is often challenging. However, it is important to identify those patients with a negligible chance of neurological recovery in order to appropriately focus care on palliation and avoid futile invasive medical treatments. Many prognostic factors are quoted at the bedside that are often supported by a very limited evidence base. Since the adoption of therapeutic hypothermia and targeted temperature management, the issue has been highlighted and consensus reviews provided to guide best practice.

Somatosensory evoked potentials monitor the brain response to peripheral nerve stimulation: the N20 potential evoked in the somatosensory cortex following median nerve stimulation has consistently demonstrated a false-positive rate of 0% when bilaterally absent at days 1-3 post-arrest. The GCS is particularly limited in this role and has little supporting evidence of validity in isolation, especially in the early stages post-cardiac arrest. Likewise, pupillary reactions are an insensitive tool for prediction of futility in the early stages post-cardiac arrest especially in the era of targeted temperature management.

Myoclonic status epilepticus is consistently associated with a poor prognosis regardless of temperature management, although it must be noted that this clinical sign will be rendered useless in patients paralysed to prevent shivering in therapeutic hypothermia.

CT imaging can be suggestive regarding grey/white matter differentiation but has no supporting evidence for its use in the prognosis post-cardiac arrest. Several scoring systems have been developed to attempt the prediction of outcome, including the Brain Arrest Neurological Outcome Scale (BrANOS). Caveats include the lack of validation in patients undergoing targeted temperature management.

1.   Tiainen M, Kovala TT, Takkunen OS, *et al.* Somatosensory and brainstem auditory evoked potentials in cardiac arrest patients treated with hypothermia. *Crit Care Med* 2005; 33: 1736-40.
2.   Zandbergen EG, de Haan RJ, Stoutenbeek CP, *et al.* Systematic review of early prediction of poor outcome in anoxic-ischaemic coma. *Lancet* 1998; 352: 1808-12.
3.   Torbey MT, Geocadin R, Bhardwaj A. Brain arrest neurological outcome scale (BrANOS): predicting mortality and severe disability following cardiac arrest. *Resuscitation* 2004; 63: 55-63.
4.   Temple A, Porter R. Predicting neurological outcome and survival after cardiac arrest. *Contin Educ Anaesth Crit Care Pain* 2012; 6: 1-5.

24   F, F, F, T, T

The European Centre for Disease Prevention and Control and the Center for Disease Control and Prevention have created a standardised international terminology with which to describe acquired resistance profiles for common bacteria responsible for healthcare-associated infections, which are also prone to multidrug resistance. Multidrug resistance (MDR) is defined as acquired non-susceptibility to at least one agent in three or more antimicrobial categories. Extensively drug-resistant (XDR) is defined as non-susceptibility to at least one agent in all but two or fewer antimicrobial categories, and pandrug resistance (PDR) is defined as non-susceptibility to all agents in all antimicrobial categories. Methicillin-resistant *Staphylococcus aureus* strains are all resistant to β-lactams, penicillins, cephalosporins and carbapenems. Healthcare-acquired strains of MRSA are MDR, i.e. they are also resistant to other classes of antibiotics such as macrolides and quinolones. Community-associated strains of MRSA (CA-MRSA) carry the Panton-Valentine leukocidin virulence factor. CA-MRSA is emerging in patients (usually children and young adults) without the traditional risk factors, causes mainly skin and soft tissue infection and, less frequently, necrotising pneumonia, and is usually susceptible to multiple classes of antimicrobials. Tigecycline is a glycylcycline antibiotic with activity against MRSA and Gram-negative bacteria (except notably *Pseudomonas aeruginosa*), including MDR strains, and *Acinetobacter baumannii*. Linezolid is an oxazolidinone which works by inhibiting microbial protein synthesis. It has 100% oral bioavailability and is a suitable alterative to vancomycin for the treatment of MRSA.

1. Magiorakos AP, Srinivasan A, Carey RB, *et al*. Multidrug-resistant, extensively drug-resistant and pandrug-resistant bacteria: an international expert proposal for interim standard definitions for acquired resistance. *Clin Microbiol Infect* 2012; 18(3): 268-81.

25 F, F, F, T, T

Acute liver failure (ALF) is a rare but multisystem condition of various aetiologies. In the developed world, paracetamol overdose is the most common cause of ALF; however, worldwide, viral aetiologies such as hepatitis A, B and E and seronegative hepatitis are more prevalent. The management of such patients on the ICU may increase their survival chances before the next steps (e.g. liver transplantation) are taken.

The diagnosis of ALF is made using the specific criteria listed below in Table 3.3. Please note however that the clinical picture is often dominated by coagulopathy and encephalopathy.

> **Table 3.3.** Clinical features required for the diagnosis of acute liver failure.

- Absence of chronic liver disease
- Acute hepatitis shown by elevation in aspartate transaminase (AST)/alanine transaminase (ALT) accompanied by elevation in the INR >1.5
- Any degree of mental alteration (encephalopathy)
- Illness less than 26 weeks' duration (ALF can be further subdivided into hyperacute, acute and subacute with an onset time from the initial insult of under 7 days, 28 days and 26 weeks, respectively)

1. Trotter JF. Practical management of acute liver failure in the intensive care unit. *Curr Opin Crit Care* 2009; 15: 163-7.

26   F, F, T, T, F

Care of the post-cardiac arrest syndrome has shifted over the last decade from individual organ support to aggressive control of the inflammatory response and early definitive intervention.

As well as patients presenting with ST elevation myocardial infarction (MI), there is emerging evidence that patients without definitive changes associated with MI on the ECG still have a high rate of coronary occlusion on angiography. There is some suggestion of benefit for early cardiac catheterisation to reduce the risk of death in this cohort; however, randomised controlled trial evidence to support this strategy is lacking. Hyperoxia has been noted to paradoxically increase the risk of death in large cohort studies. As such, the current recommendations focus on avoidance and achieving normoxia when possible.

Temperature management has been the subject of much debate recently, with a large trial suggesting no difference in outcome between post-cardiac arrest patients cooled to 33°C versus 36°C. Although this suggests that therapeutic hypothermia may be of limited benefit, there is still convincing overall evidence that targeted temperature management and avoidance of hyperthermia improves outcomes when compared to patients who are not temperature managed. Glycaemic control is recommended nationally and internationally in consensus documents. β-blockade has no supporting role at present.

1. Hollenbeck RD, McPherson JA, Mooney MR, *et al.* Early cardiac catheterization is associated with improved survival in comatose survivors of cardiac arrest without STEMI. *Resuscitation* 2013; 85(1): 88-95.
2. Kilgannon JH, Jones AE, Shapiro NI, *et al.* Association between arterial hyperoxia following resuscitation from cardiac arrest and in-hospital mortality *JAMA* 2010; 303(21): 2165-71.
3. Nielsen N, Wetterslev J, Cronberg T, *et al.* Targeted temperature management at 33 degrees Celsius versus 36 degrees Celsius after cardiac arrest. *New Engl J Med* 2013; 369: 2197-206.
4. Stub D, Bernard S, Duffy SJ, Kaye DM. Post cardiac arrest syndrome: a review of therapeutic strategies. *Circulation* 2011; 123: 1428-35.

27 F, T, F, F, T

Oxygen saturations are measured using a spectrophotometric technique, which involves shining radiation through a sample and measuring the quantity of radiation absorbed. Two light-emitting diodes are used that emit light at different wavelengths — red and infrared. These two wavelengths are used because haemoglobin and oxyhaemoglobin have different absorption spectra at these particular wavelengths. The accuracy of commercially available oximeters differs widely, but oximeters have a mean difference (bias) of <2% and a standard deviation (precision) of <3% when SpO_2 is 90% or above. Accuracy deteriorates when SpO_2 falls to 80% or less. Oximeters have a number of limitations which may lead to inaccurate readings. Pulse oximeters tend to read around 85% in the presence of elevated levels of methaemoglobin and therefore usually underestimate the oxyhaemoglobin saturation. As pulse oximeters employ only two wavelengths of light, they can distinguish only two substances. In the presence of elevated carboxyhaemoglobin levels, oximetry consistently overestimates the true SaO_2. Severe hyperbilirubinaemia (mean bilirubin 30.6mg/dL [523.26mmol/L]) does not affect the accuracy of pulse oximetry.

1. Jubran A. Pulse oximetry. *Crit Care* 1999; 3: R11-7.

28 T, F, T, F, F

APACHE II, a severity-of-disease classification system, is one of several ICU scoring systems. It is applied within 24 hours of admission of a patient to an ICU and delivers an integer score from 0 to 71; higher scores correspond to more severe disease and a higher mortality risk.

The point score is calculated from 12 routine physiological measurements (listed below in Table 3.4).

Table 3.4. APACHE II classification — physiological variables.

1.	Age
2.	Temperature (rectal)
3.	Mean arterial pressure
4.	pH arterial
5.	Heart rate
6.	Respiratory rate
7.	Sodium (serum)
8.	Potassium (serum)
9.	Creatinine
10.	Haematocrit
11.	White blood cell count
12.	Glasgow Coma Scale

1.   Bouch DC, Thompson JP. Severity scoring systems in the critically ill. *Contin Educ Anaesth Crit Care Pain* 2008; 8(5): 181-5.
2.   Knaus WA, Draper EA, Wagner DP, Zimmerman JE. APACHE - Acute Physiology and Chronic Health Evaluation: a severity of disease classification system. *Crit Care Med* 1985; 13: 818-29.

29   T, T, F, F, F

In the case of an externally draining pancreatic fistula there is a loss of bicarbonate-rich fluid externally. Excessive infusion of normal saline causes a relative hyperchloraemia with a resultant fall in the strong ion difference causing a metabolic acidosis. In the case of a urinary diversion, urinary chloride ions are exchanged across the bowel wall for bicarbonate ions which are then lost from the circulation. In all these examples the anion gap is normal. In renal failure there is a failure to excrete unmeasured organic acids, and in lactic acidosis there is excessive lactic acid production through anaerobic metabolism; both cause a raised anion gap metabolic acidosis.

1.   http://www.ccmtutorials.com/renal/Acid%20Base%20Balance%20in%20Critical%20Care%20Medicine-NELIGAN.pdf (accessed 22nd December 2014).

30   T, T, T, T, F

The intra-aortic balloon pump (IABP) is inserted percutaneously into the femoral artery (or subclavian, axillary, brachial or iliac arteries). The catheter is advanced under fluoroscopic guidance, into the descending aorta, with its tip approximately 2-3cm distal to the origin of the subclavian artery (at the level of the carina). Malpositioning can cause upper limb, cerebral or renal compromise (due to the obstruction of the brachiocephalic, common carotid and renal arteries, respectively), by the tip of the IABP. Correct placement of the tip of the central venous catheter is important for accurate measurement of central venous pressure. The central venous catheter should lie along the long axis of the vessel with the tip in the superior vena cava (SVC) or at the junction of the SVC and right atrium, outside the pericardial reflection. The pericardium lies below the level of the carina, therefore a position at the carina is satisfactory. Endotracheal tube position should be confirmed with a chest radiograph. A correctly placed endotracheal tube lies at the level of the mid-trachea, about 5-6cm above the carina. This allows for flexion and extension of the head without inadvertent extubation or bronchial intubation. The nasogastric tube must be seen to clearly bisect the carina or bronchi, cross the diaphragm in the midline, have a tip clearly visible below the left hemi-diaphragm and avoid the contours of the bronchi. Placement of a tracheostomy tube cannot be inferred from a chest radiograph; visual inspection with a flexible fibreoptic scope is advocated.

1. Krishna M, Zacharowski K. Principles of intra-aortic balloon pump counterpulsation. *Contin Educ Anaesth Crit Care Pain* 2009; 9(1): 24-8.
2. Khan AN, Al-Jahdali H, Al-Ghanem S, Gouda A. Reading chest radiographs in the critically ill (Part I): normal chest radiographic appearance, instrumentation and complications from instrumentation. *Ann Thorac Med* 2009; 4(2): 75-87.
3. Waldmann C, Soni N, Rhodes A. *Oxford Desk Reference Critical Care*. Oxford, UK: Oxford University Press, 2008.
4. National Patient Safety Agency. Patient Safety Alert NPSA/2011/PSA001. Reducing the harm caused by misplaced nasogastric feeding tubes in adults, children and infants. London, UK: NPSA, 2011.

31   F, T, F, F, F

Lactic acidosis is the most common cause of metabolic acidosis. It is associated with an elevated anion gap and a plasma lactate concentration above 4mmol/L.

The anion gap is calculated as follows:

$$([Na^+] + [K^+]) - ([Cl^-] + [HCO_3^-])$$

A normal anion gap is <11mEq/L.

Lactic acid is derived from the metabolism of pyruvic acid; this reaction is catalysed by lactate dehydrogenase and involves the conversion of nicotinamide adenine dinucleotide (reduced form) (NADH) into nicotinamide adenine dinucleotide (oxidized form) (NAD+). Normal subjects produce 15-20mmol/kg of lactic acid per day. Lactate is cleared mainly by the liver (around 80%) with a contribution from the kidneys (10-20%) and skeletal muscle.

There is little difference between venous and arterial blood lactate concentrations and measurement of either is a suitable guide to the adequacy of fluid resuscitation.

There are two types of lactic acidosis (Cohen & Woods classification). Type A lactic acidosis occurs secondary to marked tissue hypoperfusion with excessive anaerobic metabolism and thus lactate production. Type B lactic acidosis is unrelated to systemic hypoperfusion and may be due to a variety of causes including drugs, diabetes mellitus, malignancy, regional ischaemia and mitochondrial dysfunction.

1.   Kraut JA, Madias NE. Lactic acidosis. *New Engl J Med* 2014; 371: 2309-19.

32   F, F, T, F, T

Donation after cardiac death (DCD) involves a planned and coordinated approach to withdrawal of care, with the intent to retrieve organs immediately following the confirmation of death. As such the warm ischaemic time (during which inadequate oxygenation or perfusion to the organs exists) is increased in comparison to donation after brainstem death. Warm ischaemia time is defined as the time between onset of asystole and cold perfusion of the organs, and a degree of warm ischaemia time is inevitable in DCD patients. A more useful concept is that of functional warm ischaemia time, which can be defined as beginning when the donor's systolic arterial pressure is <50mmHg or SpO_2 <70%, ending with cold perfusion of the organs.

The lungs tolerate absent circulation well, provided they remain inflated with oxygen and as such may be the ideal organ for DCD. The procedure is in its infancy but gaining acceptance. The modified Maastricht classification system groups potential DCD patients into five categories, of which III is awaiting cardiac arrest and IV is cardiac arrest in a brainstem dead donor. Other groups are all uncontrolled DCD patients.

Current UK guidance suggests confirmation of death after 5 minutes of continued cardiorespiratory arrest. A further 5-minute grace period is recommended after pronouncement of death prior to commencement of organ retrieval. This is known cumulatively as the 10-minute 'hands off' time and has the function of ensuring irreversible brainstem death (in addition to cardiac death) prior to any attempt at retrieval.

With regard to approach, there is evidence to suggest that an approach consisting solely of a resident Senior Nurse for Organ Donation (SNOD) or similar professional maximises positive consent/authorisation, although the level of evidence is limited.

1. Kootstra G, Daemen JHC, Oomen APA. Categories of non-heartbeating donors. *Transpl Proc* 1995; 27: 2893-4.
2. http://www.bts.org.uk/Documents/Guidelines/Active/DCD%20for%20BTS%20and%20ICS%20FINAL.pdf (accessed 26th February 2015).
3. Vincent A, Logan L. Consent for organ donation. *Br J Anaesth* 2012; 108(Suppl 1): i80-7.

33 T, F, T, T, F

The intra-arterial blood pressure (IABP) measuring system consists of a column of fluid directly connecting the arterial tree to a pressure transducer. The pressure waveform is transmitted via the column of fluid, to a pressure transducer where it is converted into an electrical signal. This electrical signal is then processed, amplified and converted into a visual display by a microprocessor. Short, narrow, parallel-sided cannulae are used to reduce the risk of arterial thrombus formation. Small-diameter cannulas (20-22G) are used to decrease the risk of thrombus formation but this may increase damping of the system. A bag of either 0.9% saline or heparinised 0.9% saline is pressurised to 300mmHg and attached to the fluid-filled tubing via a flushing system. This allows a slow infusion of fluid at a rate of about 2-4ml/hr to maintain the patency of the cannula.

The natural frequency of the system is the frequency at which it oscillates freely. If the natural frequency of the IABP system lies close to the frequency of any of the sine wave components of the arterial waveform, then the system will resonate, causing distortion of the signal. Reducing the length of the cannula or tubing will increase the natural frequency of the system. Anything that reduces energy in an oscillating system will reduce the amplitude of the oscillations; this is 'damping'. The addition of three-way taps, bubbles and clots, vasospasm, kinks and narrow, long or compliant tubing will cause damping which may be excessive (overdamping). Overdamping causes an under-reading of systolic blood pressure and an over-reading of diastolic blood pressure, but little effect on the mean blood pressure.

For a pressure transducer to read accurately, atmospheric pressure must be discounted from the pressure measurement. This is done by exposing the transducer to atmospheric pressure and calibrating the pressure reading to zero. At this point, the level of the transducer is not important. However, the pressure transducer must be set at the level of the patient's heart, at the 4th intercostal space, in the mid-axillary line to measure the blood pressure correctly.

1. World Federation of Societies of Anaesthesiologists. Jones A, Pratt O. Physical principles of intra-arterial blood pressure measurement. Anaesthesia Tutorial of the Week 137, 2009. www.aagbi.org/education/educational-resources/tutorial-week (accessed 25th August 2014).

34   F, T, F, T, F

X-rays are of limited help in distinguishing between the various types of joint arthropathies but may show chondrocalcinosis. However, joint aspiration and examination of the synovial fluid is important and can help determine the cause of a monoarthritis. A white cell count of $>25,000/mm^3$ with more than 90% neutrophils aspirated from the joint is a strong predictor of bacterial arthritis. In such circumstances, antibiotic treatment should be commenced pending the results of the Gram stain and culture. The Gram stain of an aspirate has a high positive predictive value but a low negative predictive value for ruling in or out septic arthritis. The joint should be aspirated as soon as possible but there is no defined time period for this. Fever is common in septic arthritis but has a sensitivity of only 57%, so its absence does not exclude the diagnosis. Blood inflammatory markers are usually raised in septic arthritis so they are sensitive, but may be raised for numerous reasons (so non-specific). This is especially so if the patient has coexisting and predisposing conditions such as rheumatoid arthritis or other connective tissue diseases. Orthopaedic input should be obtained without delay as once the diagnosis is confirmed on Gram stain and culture, the joint should be washed out as soon as possible to avoid destruction.

1.   Margaretten ME, Kohwles J, Moore D, *et al.* Does this adult patient have septic arthritis? *JAMA* 2007; 297(13): 1478-88.
2.   Cunningham G, Seghrouchni K, Ruffieux E, *et al.* Gram and acridine orange staining for diagnosis of septic arthritis in different patient populations. *Int Orthop* 2014; 36(8): 1283-90.

35   T, T, T, T, F

The diagnosis of death following irreversible cessation of brainstem function can provide clarity to relatives of the patient with profound neurological insult and can facilitate the practice of 'heart beating' donation after brainstem death. In order to undertake brainstem testing, there should be no doubt that the patient's condition is due to irreversible brain damage of known aetiology. In addition, all potentially reversible causes of coma should be considered and excluded as necessary.

Multiple physiological preconditions should be satisfied prior to testing, including normothermia (temperature >34°C) and the exclusion of any reversible circulatory, metabolic and endocrine disturbances that may be contributing towards unconsciousness. These disturbances include pH <7.35, serum potassium <2mmol/L, glucose level <3mmol/L, sodium >160mmol/L or <115mmol/L, magnesium >3.0mmol/L and others.

Therapeutic drug monitoring should be considered if available, or there is concern about a residual drug effect of sedation interfering with conscious level. It is recommended that brainstem testing should not be undertaken if thiopentone levels are >5mg/L or midazolam levels are >10µg/L. In the absence of available drug monitoring and when concern persists, ancillary tests are recommended.

1.   Academy of Medical Royal Colleges. A code of practice for the diagnosis and confirmation of death. London, UK: Academy of Medical Royal Colleges, 2008.

36 T, T, T, F, T

Virchow's triad identifies hypercoagulability, vessel wall injury and stasis as the pathogenic basis for thrombosis. Approximately 25% of patients with venous thromboembolism have no apparent provoking risk factor, 50% have a temporary provoking risk factor and 25% have cancer. Intrinsic risk factors for pulmonary embolism include previous venous thromboembolism, age >70 years and an inherited hypercoagulable state. Acquired factors include obesity, pregnancy and the puerperium, oestrogen therapy, prolonged immobility, malignancy, cancer chemotherapy, major or lower limb trauma, lower limb orthopaedic surgery, general anaesthesia for >30 minutes, heparin-induced thrombocytopaenia and antiphospholipid antibodies. Immune thrombocytopaenia, formerly known as idiopathic thrombocytopaenic purpura, is an autoimmune disorder characterised by thrombocytopaenia and an increased risk of mucocutaneous bleeding. It is a diagnosis of exclusion.

1. Lapner AT, Kearon C. Clinical Review. Diagnosis and management of pulmonary embolism. *Br Med J* 2013; 346: f757.
2. Thota S, Kistangari G, Daw H, Spiro T. Immune thrombocytopaenia in adults: an update. *Cleveland Clinic Journal of Medicine* 2012; 79(9): 641-50.

37 F, T, F, F, F

Serotonin syndrome is a condition which presents very acutely, unlike neuroleptic malignant syndrome (NMS) which can present over several days. It is characterised as a triad of altered mental status such as confusion and hallucinations, autonomic instability presenting as tachycardia, hyperthermia and labile blood pressure, and neuromuscular signs including hyperreflexia, clonus and myoclonus. A variety of medications can be precipitants, including tricyclic antidepressants, monoamine oxidase inhibitors, lithium, fentanyl, sodium valproate and ondansetron, as well as recreational drugs such as sympathomimetics which are often abused. It is a dose-related condition as opposed to NMS

Paper 3 Answers

which is an idiosyncratic drug reaction to dopamine antagonists and presents with extrapyramidal signs, fluctuating consciousness and autonomic instability. Cyproheptadine is in fact a treatment of the condition as it is a serotonin antagonist.

1.   Boyer EW, Shannon M. The serotonin syndrome. *New Engl J Med* 2005; 352: 1112-20.

38   T, F, T, T, F

Thromboelastography (TEG®) is a novel point-of-care viscoelastic haemostatic assay that provides rapid information on the process of whole blood clot formation. It provides valuable data on platelet interaction and function, fibrinolysis and general clot formation and stability. It has been widely used in cardiothoracic surgery for some time and with increasing evidence of its effect in reducing blood product use, it is being trialled in other clinical situations.

TEG® seeks to assess the physical properties of the clot in whole blood. The test is performed by collection of whole blood, which is then transferred to a container (cup) in which a pin is suspended by a torsion wire. Rotation is incurred and the elasticity/strength of the developing clot affects the rotation of the pin. These data are charted in graphical and numeric form to give an overview of clot formation and function.

With regard to the output, TEG® produces a variety of discrete intervals. Reaction time, or R-time, is measured as the time from the start of the test to initial fibrin formation/clot initiation. Kinetics, or K-time, are measured as the time to achieve a certain degree of clot strength. The α-angle measures the slope between R and K, and as such the speed at which fibrin build-up and cross-linking occurs. Maximal amplitude (MA) represents the final peak stability of the clot. Lysis at 30 minutes (LY30) looks for the change in amplitude at 30 minutes as a representation of fibrinolysis. When this is enhanced, the entire trace may well have returned to baseline suggesting complete clot destruction within 30 minutes.

While there is reasonable evidence to support a reduction in product use with TEG® in surgical care, the highest level of evidence in trauma is currently cohort studies only. Further evidence is needed before this can be regarded as a standard of care.

1.   Ganter MT, Hofer CK. Coagulation monitoring: current techniques and clinical use of viscoelastic point-of-care coagulation devices. *Anesth Analg* 2008; 106(5): 1366-75.
2.   Afshari A, Wikkelsø A, Brok J, *et al.* Thrombelastography (TEG) or thromboelastometry (ROTEM) to monitor haemotherapy versus usual care in patients with massive transfusion. *Cochrane Database Syst Rev* 2011; 3: CD007871.

39   T, F, F, T, F

Low-molecular-weight heparin (LMWH) can be partially reversed with protamine. In the acutely bleeding patient, administration of blood and blood products should be informed by laboratory results and near-patient testing, but led by the clinical situation. Guidelines vary, but the 2013 European trauma guideline suggests maintaining a platelet count ≥ 100 x 10^9/L in cases of traumatic bleeding with a fibrinogen level of 1.5-2g/L. Tranexamic acid inhibits fibrinolysis by blocking the lysine binding sites on plasminogen. The CRASH-2 trial was a randomised controlled trial which enrolled 20,211 adult trauma patients with, or at risk of, significant bleeding. A loading dose of 1g tranexamic acid was given over 10 minutes, then a further 1g was infused over 8 hours. All-cause mortality, and the risk of death due to bleeding, was significantly reduced in the treatment group. Early treatment (1 hour or less from injury), and treatment delivered between 1 and 3 hours post-injury significantly reduced the risk of death due to bleeding but treatment given after 3 hours was associated with an increased risk of death due to bleeding and therefore is not recommended.

Group O RhD negative is the blood group of choice in an emergency where the clinical need is immediate. However, overdependence on group O RhD negative red cells may have an adverse impact on local and national blood stock management and it is considered acceptable to give O RhD positive red cells to male patients in this situation. Patients with massive haemorrhage are also prothrombotic and at increased risk of thromboembolic disease, so thromboprophylaxis should be started early following achievement of haemostasis (assuming no intracranial bleeding has occurred).

1.   Association of Anaesthetists of Great Britain and Ireland. Blood transfusion and the anaesthetist: management of massive haemorrhage. *Anaesthesia* 2010; 65: 1153-61.
2.   CRASH-2 trial collaborators. Effects of tranexamic acid on death, vascular occlusive events, and blood transfusion in trauma patients with significant haemorrhage (CRASH-2): a randomised, placebo-controlled trial. *Lancet* 2010; 376: 23-32.
3.   CRASH-2 collaborators. The importance of early treatment with tranexamic acid in bleeding trauma patients: an exploratory analysis of the CRASH-2 randomised controlled trial. *Lancet* 2011; 377(9771): 1096-101.
4.   Spahn DR, Bouillon B, Cerny V, *et al.* Management of bleeding and coagulopathy following major trauma: an updated European guideline. *Crit Care* 2013; 17: R76.

40   F, F, F, T, F

Some of these devices are permanent and some are removable. They do reduce the incidence of a further pulmonary embolism (PE) but they also increase the risk of deep vein thrombosis. They have not shown to improve long-term survival, although they do reduce the incidence of PE. The majority of vena cava filters are non-ferromagnetic and therefore compatible with magnetic resonance imaging (MRI). Prophylactic placement is a weak indication; the strongest evidence to support placement of a filter is in cases of proven venous thromboembolism (VTE) where anticoagulation is contraindicated, and in patients with recurrent VTE despite therapeutic anticoagulation.

1.   Tapson VF. Acute pulmonary embolism. *New Engl J Med* 2008; 358(10): 1037-52.

41   T, F, F, T, T

Death after cardiorespiratory death is diagnosed by a registered medical practitioner, or other appropriately trained and qualified individual, and confirms the irreversible cessation of neurological (pupillary), cardiac and respiratory activity. This is performed by observation for a minimum of 5 minutes confirming the absence of respiratory effort and the absence of heart sounds on auscultation. After 5 minutes the absence of pupillary response to light and the absence of any motor response to supra-orbital pressure must be confirmed. The diagnosis of death is made once all these criteria are fulfilled. In the hospital setting, the absence of mechanical cardiac function can be confirmed by asystole on a continuous ECG display, the absence of pulsatile flow using direct intra-arterial pressure monitoring or the absence of contractile activity using echocardiography.

Brainstem death testing can only be undertaken when there is a known aetiology of irreversible brain damage and potentially reversible causes of coma are excluded; this includes iatrogenic causes and physiological disturbances of normal body homeostasis. It is recommended that core temperature should be greater than 34°C at the time of testing and serum potassium levels should be greater than 2mmol/L. In cases of proven or suspected high spinal injury, the apnoea test becomes invalid. Cessation of brainstem function can be established only by confirming the absence of other brainstem reflexes and using ancillary investigations, including tests of blood flow in the larger cerebral arteries, brain tissue perfusion and neurophysiology studies.

1. Academy of Medical Royal Colleges. A code of practice for the diagnosis and confirmation of death. London, UK: Academy of Medical Royal Colleges, 2008.

42   F, T, F, T, F

Hyponatraemia is defined as a serum sodium concentration of less than 135mmol/L and is the most common disorder of body fluid and electrolyte balance encountered in clinical practice. Severe symptoms of hyponatraemia are caused by brain oedema and increased intracranial pressure. It takes the brain approximately 24-48 hours to move osmotically active particles between the intracellular and extracellular compartments to restore brain volume, hence, a 48-hour threshold to distinguish acute (<48 hours) from chronic (>48 hours) hyponatraemia. SIADH occurs due to the increased release of vasopressin by the pituitary gland or from ectopic production. It does lead to hypotonic hyponatraemia with normal extracellular fluid volume. When correcting hyponatraemia, the increase in serum sodium concentration during the first 24 hours should be limited to

0.5mmol/L/hr. Patients with severe symptoms of hyponatraemia (vomiting, cardiorespiratory distress, abnormal or deep somnolence, seizures and coma) require urgent treatment. Prompt IV infusion of 150-300ml 3% saline over 20 minutes is recommended. Serum sodium concentration should be retested and further treatment tailored accordingly, aiming for an increase of 5mmol/L or resolution of symptoms. Following correction of serum hyponatraemia it may take some time for the brain to recover due to equilibration across the blood brain barrier; therefore, severe symptoms may not resolve immediately.

1.   Spasovski G, Vanholder R, Allolio B, et al. Clinical practice guideline on diagnosis and treatment of hyponatraemia. Eur J Endocrinol 2014; 170: G1-47.

43   F, F, F, T, F

Delirium in critically ill patients is a very common occurrence, with between 60% and 80% of ventilated patients developing this. Delirium is defined as a disturbance of consciousness and a change in cognition that develops over a relatively short duration. The majority of critically ill patients with delirium have either the hypoactive form or a mixed picture where they fluctuate between hyperactivity and hypoactivity. Patients with hypoactive delirium are most commonly under-diagnosed. They often wake up from sedation peacefully, nod and say yes to all questions.

Some risk factors cannot be altered such as old age, alcoholism, smoking, visual and/or hearing impairment, previous cognitive impairment, and depression. Strategies used in the non-ICU setting include continual orientation of patients, addressing visual and hearing impairments, early mobilisation, reduction of noise/stimuli and non-pharmacological sleep protocols. Iatrogenic factors can precipitate delirium and are common in the ICU: medication, sleep disturbance, and poor mobilisation.

The use of sedation scoring systems may reduce the risk of delirium. Daily sedation holds and sedation scoring are recommended, as they allow dose titration on an individual patient basis. The evidence for an association between opioids and delirium is less strong than that for benzodiazepines. Protocols that use intermittent boluses of drugs rather than continuous infusions may improve a number of outcomes including delirium.

The Confusion Assessment Method - Intensive Care Unit (CAM-ICU) test is derived from the confusion assessment method, and is designed to be used to assess patients receiving ventilator support. It has a high sensitivity (93-100%) and specificity (89-100%). The test is also simple and can be performed by all ICU staff. Delirium is diagnosed based on the assessment of four features. A 'CAM-ICU positive' (i.e. delirium present) score requires evidence of both a fluctuating mental state and evidence of inattention, together with the presence of either a sedation score other than alert and calm, or evidence of disorganised thinking.

Multiple studies have shown an association between sedative drugs and delirium, with benzodiazepines being the most strongly associated. Antipsychotics (specifically haloperidol and olanzapine) are the most effective pharmacological treatment.

1. King J, Gratrix A. Delirium in intensive care. *Contin Educ Anaesth Crit Care Pain* 2009: 9(5): 144-7.
2. http://www.icudelirium.org/docs/CAM_ICU_worksheet.pdf (accessed 18th September 2014).

44   T, F, F, F, T

Adult tracheostomy emergencies are uncommon, but carry a high risk of morbidity and mortality. Patients on the intensive care unit are particularly vulnerable to complications and often managed in an arena where specific surgical expertise is lacking. Much work has been undertaken recently on the management of, and complications with, tracheostomies on the intensive care unit, including a national report, multidisciplinary project initiative and consensus guideline.

The UK National Tracheostomy Safety Project contains readily accessible guidelines for a stepwise approach to the management of a tracheostomy critical incident. An ABCDE approach is supported, with particular emphasis on look, listen and feel at both the mouth and stoma for evidence of airflow and explicit use of waveform capnography. Oxygen should be applied early as stated. Most inner tubes are best removed early to exclude physical obstruction unless there is a specific dependent connection.

Following these measures, attempts to pass a suction catheter should be instigated, with the cuff only deflated if first attempts fail. The trachestomy should be removed early and oral intubation attempted (where feasible) if the catheter cannot be passed or if the patient continues to deteriorate despite attempted intervention. A paediatric facemask/LMA applied to the stoma or standard oral airway manoeuvres with the stoma occluded are recommended as primary emergency oxygenation strategies.

1. Wilkinson KA, Martin IC, Freeth H, et al. On the right trach? A review of the care received by patients who underwent a tracheostomy. National Confidential Enquiry into Patient Outcome and Death (NCEPOD), 2014. www.ncepod.org.uk/2014report1/downloads/On%20the%20Right%20Trach_FullReport.pdf (accessed 22nd January 2015).
2. http://www.tracheostomy.org.uk/Templates/Home.html (accessed 17th July 2014).
3. McGrath BA, Bates L, Atkinson D, Moore JA. Multidisciplinary guidelines for the management of tracheostomy and laryngectomy airway emergencies. Anaesthesia 2012; 67: 1025-41.

45 F, F, T, T, F

The most common presentation of pulmonary hypertension is with progressive breathlessness. As right ventricular dysfunction develops, patients can experience exertional dizziness and syncope. Pulmonary hypertension is defined at cardiac catheterisation as a mean pulmonary artery pressure (MPAP) of 25mmHg or more at rest. Echocardiography measures systolic pulmonary artery pressure and therefore cannot be used to make the diagnosis. Causes of pulmonary hypertension can be subdivided into pulmonary arterial hypertension, pulmonary hypertension owing to left heart disease, pulmonary hypertension owing to lung disease or hypoxia (including sleep disordered breathing), chronic thromboembolic pulmonary hypertension and those with an unclear mechanism.

Pharmacological treatment options include: high-dose calcium channel blockade (diltiazem, nifedipine), prostanoids (prostacyclin, iloprost), endothelin receptor antagonists (bosentan, ambrisentan) and phosphodiesterase-5 inhibitors (sildenafil, tadalafil).

1. Kiely DG, Elliot CA, Sabroe I, Condliffe R. Pulmonary hypertension: diagnosis and management. *Br Med J* 2013; 346: f2028.

46 F, F, T, F, F

Normal CSF values are shown in Table 3.5 along with typical values for CNS infections.

Table 3.5. Normal CSF values along with typical values for CNS infections.

	Normal	Bacterial	Viral	TB/fungal
Opening pressure (cmH$_2$O)	5-20	>30	Normal or slightly increased	Variable
Appearance	Normal	Turbid	Clear	Fibrin web
Protein (g/L)	0.2-0.4	>1	<1	0.1-0.5
Glucose (mmol/L)	2.5-3.5	<2.2	Normal	1.6-2.5
CSF glucose:serum glucose ratio	0.6	<0.4	>0.6	<0.4
Gram stain	Normal	60-90% positive	Normal	Variable
WCC	<3	>500	<1000	100-500

Typical CSF findings in GBS are an elevated protein and normal glucose concentrations. GBS associated with HIV infection leads to pleocytosis (elevated CSF leukocytes). If the white cell count is high then it should raise concerns about another potential diagnosis. Oligoclonal bands are sensitive for demyelination processes and may be present in GBS, although monoclonal bands are a feature of myeloma.

1. Winer JB. Clinical review: Guillan-Barré syndrome. *Br Med J* 2008; 337: a671.
2. Ramrakah P, Moore K. Practical procedures. *Oxford Handbook of Acute Medicine*, 3rd ed. Oxford, UK: Oxford University Press, 2010.

47 T, T, F, F, F

Selective digestive tract decontamination (SDD) and selective oropharyngeal decontamination (SOD) have been extensively assessed within the medical literature as a method for prevention of nosocomial respiratory infection on the intensive care unit. Common regimens include the use of enteral polymyxin, amphotericin and tobramycin.

Collated evidence from systematic review articles suggest a decrease in both the risk of death and ventilator-associated pneumonia development with this therapy. Despite relatively convincing data, there continues to be a reluctance to introduce the therapy to mainstream use. Contrary to expectation, there is no current evidence to suggest that SDD or SOD lead to increased rates of clostridial infection or antibiotic resistance.

The SUDDICU (Selective Decontamination of the Digestive tract in critically ill patients treated in Intensive Care Units) project is a collective multicentre collaboration gathering evidence in support of the use of SDD in critical care, through systematic review Delphi consensus and further high-quality randomised controlled trials.

1. Liberati A, D'Amico R, Pifferi S, *et al.* Antibiotic prophylaxis to reduce respiratory tract infections and mortality in adults receiving intensive care. *Cochrane Database Syst Rev* 2009; 4: CD000022.
2. Daneman N, Sarwar S, Fowler RA, *et al.* Effect of selective decontamination on antimicrobial resistance in intensive care units: a systematic review and meta-analysis. *Lancet Infect Dis* 2013; 13(4): 328-41.

3. Cuthbertson BH, Francis J, Campbell MK, *et al.* A study on the perceived risks, benefits and barriers to the use of SDD in adult critical care units (The SuDDICU) study. *Trials* 2010; 11: 117.

48   T, F, F, F, T

For platelets to adhere to a damaged vascular surface, both fibrinogen and von Willebrand Factor (vWF) are necessary. vWF functions primarily to promote platelet adhesion to the subendothelial layers at high shear rates and, in addition, acts as a carrier molecule for Factor VIII coagulant protein in the circulation. In acquired haemophilia, autoantibodies are directed against a coagulation factor, usually Factor VIII. This is commonly associated with autoimmune disorders, drug reactions or the postpartum period. They are diagnosed in the presence of a prolonged time in the coagulation screen, which fails to correct on addition of normal plasma.

Heparin-induced thrombocytopaenia is a disorder in which a falling platelet count occurs in association with a progressive thrombotic tendency, which affects large vessels, both arterial and venous. The thrombocytopaenia is caused by a specific antibody to platelet Factor 4, which promotes platelet aggregation to initiate thrombosis. Glanzmann thrombasthenia is an autosomal recessive defect which leads to abnormalities of the GP IIb/IIIa receptor and is most often encountered in patient populations in which there is a high incidence of consanguinity. Desmopressin (DDAVP) triggers the release of vWF from Weibel-Palade bodies of vascular endothelium and therefore promotes haemostasis. It is increasingly being used to manage patients with abnormalities of primary haemostasis (especially von Willebrand disease), patients exposed to aspirin and cirrhotic patients with bleeding complications.

1. Triplett DA. Coagulation and bleeding disorders: review and update. *Clinical Chemistry* 2000; 46(8B): 1260-9.
2. Martlew VJ. Peri-operative management of patients with coagulation disorders. *Br J Anaesth* 2000; 85(3): 446-55.

49   F, F, F, T, F

The Sengstaken-Blakemore tube can be very useful in a massive upper gastrointestinal variceal haemorrhage and may help control bleeding in up to 90% of cases. However, rebleeding may occur in up to 50% of cases on deflation of the balloon. It has three ports (gastric balloon inflation, gastric aspiration, oesophageal balloon inflation), unlike the Minnesota tube which has an additional fourth port to enable aspiration of the oesophagus, thereby reducing aspiration risk. Although some authorities advocate storing the tube in a fridge there is no evidence that this improves insertion or efficacy.

It is inserted via the oral or nasal route. Pre-insertion checks include inflating the gastric and oesophageal balloon. Once inserted to a distance of 55cm from incisors, the gastric balloon is inflated with either saline or air with a volume as indicated on each port. Sometimes contrast is used in this inflation to allow a better idea of position on chest X-ray exam.

The tube is then placed on traction to keep the gastric balloon abutting the gastro-oesophageal junction and tamponading oesophageal varices. If the bleeding does not stop, the oesophageal balloon may need inflation, but to prevent oesophageal necrosis, this needs deflation every 4 hours for 15 minutes. It is recommended that the tube is usually removed within 36-48 hours.

1.   Waldmann C, Soni N, Rhodes A. *Oxford Desk Reference Critical Care.* Oxford, UK: Oxford University Press, 2008.

50   F, T, F, F, F

The last few years has seen the publication of several trials regarding thrombolysis in acute submassive and massive pulmonary embolism (PE). The term 'submassive' implies preserved blood pressure and peripheral perfusion but with evidence of right heart strain. As the literature emerges our understanding of risk and benefit in this challenging condition increases. At recent meta-analysis, a comparison of mortality rates for those patients managed with thrombolysis versus anticoagulation alone suggests a significant reduction in favour of thrombolysis, from 3.89% to 2.17% (number needed to treat [NNT] of 59). This figure is lower than that quoted in many registries and may reflect exclusion criteria for entry into the trials considered. Although this result was significant, the high NNT reminds us that the overall mortality without thrombolysis is actually quite low. Coupled to this high NNT is the unfortunate association with major bleeding. This is markedly increased with thrombolysis in those patients over the age of 65, with an event rate approaching 13% and an odds ratio of 3.10 (95% CI 2.10-4.56) when compared to anticoagulation alone. Interestingly, no significant increase in major bleeding rates is reported with thrombolysis in the age group <65.

Most of the evidence concerning the efficacy of thrombolysis for pulmonary embolism concerns peripherally administered thrombolytic agents; while some studies have examined catheter-directed thrombolysis, this is not a current standard of care. The presence of right ventricular dysfuction is a marker of haemodynamic compromise that partly defines submassive pulmonary embolism; in its absence thrombolysis should not generally be administered as the degree of haemodynamic disturbance (and therefore clinical risk of mortality) is not high enough to justify the risks of the therapy (number needed to harm of 18 for major bleeding).

Half standard dose thrombolysis is an emerging therapy supported by the MOPETT (Moderate Pulmonary Embolism Treated with Thrombolysis) trial data. This study recently suggested a benefit in reduction of pulmonary hypertension after >2 years of follow-up and a non-significant trend towards reduced early mortality with low-dose thrombolytics in submassive PE. In addition, no increase in the rate of major bleeding was seen between groups. However, these are data from a single-centre trial in need of validation and unsuitable for general recommendation at present.

Overall, there is ongoing debate over the efficacy of thrombolysis in patients with submassive pulmonary embolism, and thrombolysis is not at present advocated for such patients in the most recent European guidelines.

Paper 3 Answers

1.   Chatterjee S, Chakraborty A, Weinberg I, *et al*. Thrombolysis for pulmonary embolism and risk of all-cause mortality, major bleeding, and intracranial hemorrhage: a meta-analysis. *JAMA* 2014; 311(23): 2414-21.
2.   Sharifi M, Bay C, Skrocki L. Moderate pulmonary embolism treated with thrombolytic therapy. *Am J Cardiol* 2013; 111(2): 273-7.
3.   Konstantinides SV, Torbicki A, Agnelli G, *et al*. 2014 ESC guidelines on the diagnosis and management of acute pulmonary embolism. *Eur Heart J* 2014; 35: 3033-80.

51   F, F, T, F, F

The diagnosis of acute pancreatitis (AP) is most often established by the presence of two of the following criteria: abdominal pain consistent with the disease, serum amylase and/or lipase greater than three times the upper limit of normal and/or characteristic findings from abdominal imaging. Serum lipase is more specific and remains elevated longer than amylase after disease presentation; however, lipase is also found to be elevated in a variety of non-pancreatic diseases. Serum amylase levels may remain within the normal range on admission in as many as one fifth of patients. Severe AP occurs in 15-20% of patients and is defined by the presence of persistent (fails to resolve within 48 hours) organ failure and/or death. Historically, in the absence of organ failure, local complications from pancreatitis, such as pancreatic necrosis, were also considered severe disease. CT and/or MRI of the pancreas should be reserved for patients in whom the diagnosis is unclear or who fail to improve clinically within the first 48-72 hours after hospital admission.

International consensus definition of the severity of pancreatitis suggests that organ failure present for >48 hours is required for the diagnosis of severe acute pancreatitis. Antibiotics should be given for an extrapancreatic infection but routine use of prophylactic antibiotics in patients with severe AP is not recommended. Trials have also found that the use of antibiotics in patients with sterile necrosis (to prevent the development of infected necrosis) does not confer an advantage and is therefore not recommended. In severe AP, enteral feeding is recommended to prevent infectious complications. Parenteral nutrition should be avoided, unless the enteral route is not available, not tolerated, or not meeting calorie requirements.

1.	Tenner S, Baillie J, DeWitt J, Swaroop Vege S. American College of Gastroenterology guideline: management of acute pancreatitis. *Am J Gastroenterol* 2013; 108: 1400-15.
2.	Banks PA, Bollen TL, Dervenis C, *et al.* Classification of acute pancreatitis - 2012: revision of the Atlanta classification and definitions by international consensus. *Gut* 2013; 62: 102-11.

52 T, F, T, F, T

The 'safe triangle' is the triangle bordered by the anterior border of the latissimus dorsi, the lateral border of the pectoralis major muscle, a line superior to the horizontal level of the nipple, and an apex below the axilla.

This triangle minimises the risk of damage to underlying structures such as the nearby viscera and internal mammary artery, and avoids damage to muscle and breast tissue resulting in unsightly scarring.

1.	Laws D. BTS guidelines for the insertion of a chest drain. *Thorax* 2003; 58: ii53-9.
2.	Paramasivam E, Bodenham A. Air leaks, pneumothorax and chest drains. *Contin Educ Anaesth Crit Care Pain* 2008; 8(6): 204-9.

53 F, F, F, T, T

All patients presenting within 12 hours of the onset of chest pain with a diagnosis of STEMI should be considered for reperfusion therapy. Coronary angiography (with follow-on primary PCI if indicated) is the treatment of choice, provided it can be delivered within 120 minutes of the time thrombolysis could have been given. Angiography (+/- PCI) is also indicated for patients who have residual ST-segment elevation post-fibrinolysis and those presenting greater than 12 hours after the onset of symptoms if there is evidence of ongoing myocardial ischaemia. Level of consciousness is not a factor in determining eligibility for coronary angiography, although consideration would have to be given to whether an intracranial bleed has caused the fall in GCS (which would be a contraindication). In the UK, bivalirudin in combination with aspirin and clopidogrel is recommended for the treatment of adults with STEMI undergoing primary percutaneous coronary intervention. American Heart Association guidelines specify that all patients undergoing PCI should receive a parenteral anticoagulant. Unfractionated heparin, low-molecular-weight heparin, bivalirudin, fodaparinux and argatroban are the parenteral agents used in PCI. Ticagrelor in combination with low-dose aspirin is recommended for up to 12 months as a treatment option in patients with STEMI. Ticagrelor is an oral adenosine diphosphate receptor antagonist, which inhibits platelet aggregation and thrombus formation in atherosclerotic disease. The PLATO (PLATelet inhibition and patient Outcomes) trial compared ticagrelor plus aspirin with clopidogrel plus aspirin for 12 months after an acute coronary syndrome. The relative risk of experiencing another event was 16% lower in the group treated with ticagrelor.

1. National Institute for Health and Care Excellence. Myocardial infarction with ST-segment elevation. NICE clinical guideline 167. London, UK: NICE, 2013. www.nice.org.uk (accessed 25th February 2015).
2. National Institute for Health and Care Excellence. Bivalirudin for the treatment of ST-segment-elevation myocardial infarction. NICE technology appraisal guidance 230. London, UK: NICE, 2011. www.nice.org.uk (accessed 25th February 2015).
3. Levine GN, Bates ER, Blakenship JC, et al. 2011 ACCF/AHA/SCAI guideline for percutaneous coronary intervention: a report of the American College of Cardiology Foundation/American Heart Association Task Force on Practice Guidelines and the Society for Cardiovascular Angiography and Interventions. Circulation 2011; 124: e574-651.
4. National Institute for Health and Care Excellence. Ticagrelor for the treatment of acute coronary syndromes. NICE technology appraisal guidance 236. London, UK: NICE, 2011. www.nice.org.uk (accessed 25th February 2015).

54 F, T, T, F, T

Pulmonary capillary wedge pressure (PCWP) or pulmonary artery occlusion pressure (PAOP) provides an indirect estimate of left atrial pressure (LAP). PAOP is measured by inserting a balloon-tipped, multi-lumen catheter (also known as a Swan-Ganz catheter) into a peripheral vein, advancing the catheter into the right atrium, right ventricle, pulmonary artery, and then into a branch of the pulmonary artery. The same catheter can be used to measure cardiac output by the thermodilution technique.

The pressure recorded during balloon inflation is similar to left atrial pressure because the occluded vessel and its distal branches that eventually form the pulmonary veins act as a long catheter that measures the blood pressures within the pulmonary veins and left atrium.

PAOP can be used to diagnose the severity of left ventricular failure and estimate the degree of mitral valve stenosis (large A-waves). Both of these conditions elevate LAP and therefore PAOP. These pressures are normally 8-10mmHg. Aortic valve stenosis and regurgitation, and mitral regurgitation (regurgitant V-waves) also elevate left atrial pressures and therefore PAOP. When these pressures are above 20mmHg, pulmonary oedema may often be present.

1.   Robin E, Costecalde M, Lebuffe G, Vallet B. Clinical relevance of data from the pulmonary artery catheter. *Crit Care* 2006; 10(Suppl 3): S3.

55   F, T, T, T, F

Management of burn cases in the first 24 hours reflects the risk of morbidity and mortality. Management follows an ABC approach. The burn is assessed for its percentage of total body surface area (TBSA) and the degree of burn. In adults the total burn surface area can be estimated using the 'rule of nines' but in paediatrics a Lund-Browder chart should be used due to the relative differences in body proportions. The degree of burn is now described as epidermal (skin erythema, intact skin — not part of the % area), superficial partial thickness (involvement of the epidermis and part of the papillary dermis), deep partial thickness (involvement of the epidermis and the entire papillary dermis down to the reticular dermis) and full thickness (involvement of the entire thickness of the skin and possibly subcutaneous tissue). There are many criteria for transfer to a burns centre, including those based on the percentage of burn. In patients younger than 10 years with partial-thickness, or full-thickness burns and an estimated TBSA >10%, a referral for transfer to a burn centre should be made. Burn shock resuscitation is required if the TBSA exceeds 10% (children), 15% (adults) and 10% (elderly — older than 65 years). The Parkland formula helps to calculate the fluid needs for the first 24 hours:

Volume of fluid (mL) = 4mL x Patient's body weight (kg) x TBSA (%)

50% of this volume is infused in the first 8 hours, starting from the time of injury, and the other 50% is infused during the last 16 hours of the first day. Colloids should be avoided in the first 24 hours as they can lead to prolonged tissue oedema. Burns occurring in closed areas and all burns that are affecting the head are subject to inhalational injury. Carboxyhaemoglobin levels of >20% or neurological deficits are absolute indications for hyperbaric oxygen therapy; levels >10% constitute a relative indication.

1. Alharbi Z, Piatkowski A, Dembinski R, *et al*. Treatment of burns in the first 24 hours: simple and practical guide by answering 10 questions in a step-by-step form. *World J Emerg Surg* 2012; 7(13): 1-10.
2. Alsbjoern BF. European standards. Practice guidelines for burn care. The British Burn Association. http://www.britishburnassociation.org/european-standards (accessed 17th August 2014).

56 F, T, T, T, F

The temperature of blood perfusing the hypothalamus is the reference of core body temperature. In anaesthesia and critical care, the pulmonary artery temperature is considered as the gold standard to approximate core body temperature. An oesophageal temperature probe is most accurate in the distal oesophagus; however, it loses its accuracy during thoracotomy, due to the local cooling effects of tissues. If misplaced into the upper oesophagus, the probe can be cooled by gas flow in the airways, thus decreasing its accuracy. Thermistors are semiconductors in which the resistance changes with temperature; although the change is non-linear, it can be manufactured so that it is almost linear within the working range. They are small and have rapid response times; however, they do need recalibration and are prone to drift. The frequency of infrared energy emitted by an object with temperature can be measured. Infrared tympanic thermometers measure the frequency of infrared light emitted by the tympanic membrane. The operator needs to ensure that the external auditory canal is free from wax prior to use. The Tempadot™ is an example of a thermometer which utilises heat-sensitive chemical dots. When exposed to an increase in temperature the dots melt, resulting in a change in colour. They provide a faster reaction time than mercury thermometers, taking 1 minute for an oral reading and 3 minutes for an axillary reading. Bladder temperature is determined primarily by urine flow and high flow rates are necessary for the bladder temperature to reflect core temperature. Low urinary flow makes bladder temperature difficult to interpret in relation to true core temperature.

1. Lefrant J-Y, Muller L, Emmanuel Coussaye J, *et al*. Temperature measurement in intensive care patients: comparison of urinary bladder, oesophageal, rectal, axillary, and inguinal methods versus pulmonary artery core method. *Intensive Care Med* 2003; 29: 414-8.
2. Anaesthesia UK. Temperature measurement sites. http://www.frca.co.uk/article.aspx?articleid=100352 (accessed 29th August 2014).
3. Anaesthesia UK. Temperature measurement: electrical techniques. http://www.frca.co.uk/article.aspx?articleid=100326 (accessed 29th August 2014).

57 T, F, F, F, T

MDMA is an amphetamine which can lead to toxicity due to excessive stimulation of the central nervous system. Hepatotoxicty secondary to MDMA may range from acute hepatitis to fulminant hepatic failure. This may occur as a result of acute hepatic ischaemia; however, direct effects of MDMA may also contribute. Hyponatraemia may result due to release of antidiuretic hormone, water intoxication and sodium loss through excessive sweating. Hypernatraemia and non-cardiogenic pulmonary oedema are rare. Hypertension is common as a sympathomimetic side effect, and may result in intracerebral haemorrhage in rare cases. Stroke, either ischaemic or haemorrhagic, is also a rare complication. MDMA toxicity is also associated with hyperthermia with evidence that it is dependent on environmental temperature, with increased risk of toxicity the warmer the ambient temperature. The association between hyperthermia and rhabdomyolysis, as a result of excessive muscle activity at social events combined with poor fluid intake can lead to multi-organ dysfunction.

1. Gowing LR, Henry-Edwards SM, Irvine RJ, Ali RL. The health effects of ecstasy: a literature review. *Drug Alcohol Rev* 2002; 21: 53-63.
2. Narang RK, Jadun CK, Carr B. Case report: a case of MDMA toxicity with unusual clinical and neuroradiological features. *J Intensive Care Soc* 2014; 15: 70-3.

58 T, F, T, F, T

PCO_2, total weak acid concentration (ATOT) and strong ion difference (SID) are the three independent variables in Stewart's acid-base hypothesis. This approach to understanding acid-base abnormalities emphasises the role of water dissociation and the primacy of maintaining electroneutrality. It is a useful approach to considering a variety of acid-base disturbances including hypoalbuminaemic states and the cause of a hyperchloraemic acidosis.

1.   Hubble S. Acid-base and blood gas analysis. *Anaesth Intensive Care Med* 2007; 8(11): 471-3.

59 F, F, F, T, T

There is increasing evidence that in critically ill patients, lower transfusion triggers confer a mortality benefit. The number needed to treat in a recent systematic review and meta-analysis was 33 (Salpeter *et al*). In addition to mortality, the last decade has seen fairly conclusive trial data that restrictive transfusion triggers will decrease the rate of coronary events, rebleeding, pulmonary oedema and bacterial infections for most patients. However, when interpreting the results of such studies it is important to bear in mind the heterogeneous populations involved (including paediatric and upper gastrointestinal bleeding patients in the reference quoted above).

Recent randomised controlled trials have compared restrictive to liberal transfusion in patients with acute upper GI bleeds, and those on paediatric intensive care, with results again suggesting reduced mortality and adverse outcomes in both restrictive groups. Pilot work is suggestive that patients with symptomatic coronary artery disease may benefit from higher triggers. Work is ongoing in this area.

Recombinant erythropoietin may have a role as a substitute for blood transfusion in the Jehovah's Witness patient, but sufficient time must be allowed for promotion of erythropoiesis. Following administration, the equivalent of 1 unit of blood is produced in 7 days. As such it is most effective pre-operatively and serves little purpose in the acute setting.

1. Salpeter SR, Buckley JS, Chatterjee S. Impact of more restrictive blood transfusion strategies on clinical outcomes: a meta-analysis and systematic review. *Am J Med* 2014; 127(2): 124-31.
2. Carless PA, Henry DA, Carson JL, *et al*. Transfusion thresholds and other strategies for guiding allogeneic red blood cell transfusion. *Cochrane Database Syst Rev* 2012; 10: CD002042.
3. Villanueva C, Colomo A, Bosch A, *et al*. Transfusion strategies for acute upper gastrointestinal bleeding. *New Engl J Med* 2013; 368: 11-21.
4. Lacroix J, Hébert PC, Hutchison JS, *et al*. Transfusion strategies for patients in pediatric intensive care units. *New Engl J Med* 2007; 356: 1609-19.
5. Carson JL, Brooks MM, Abbott JD, *et al*. Liberal versus restrictive transfusion thresholds for patients with symptomatic coronary artery disease. *Am Heart J* 2012; 165(6): 964-71.
6. Milligan LJ, Bellamy MC. Anaesthesia and critical care of Jehovah's Witnesses. *Contin Educ Anaesth Crit Care Pain* 2004; 4(2): 35-9.

60 T, F, T, F, T

Plateau pressure is a measure of compliance with the resistive element negated by an inspiratory hold manoeuvre. Plateau pressure therefore = P_{peak} - $P_{resistance}$. CO_2 elimination is proportional to alveolar minute volume, but total minute volume includes anatomical dead space. Hence, a low rate, deep breath strategy will eliminate more CO_2 than a high rate with lower tidal volumes. E is true as alveoli are less distended in the lung bases and therefore on a steeper part of the compliance curve.

1. West JB. *Respiratory Physiology: The Essentials*, 9th ed. Lippincott Williams & Wilkins, 2011.

61 C

The classic initial signs of malignant hyperthermia include tachycardia, hypercarbia (progressive increased end-tidal CO_2 in a ventilated patient, increasing minute volume in a spontaneously breathing patient), masseter spasm and mixed metabolic and respiratory acidosis. Of the options given, metabolic alkalosis is not a feature of MH. Hyperthermia can be a feature, but is not usually an early sign and a temperature of 38.5°C in a patient with appendicitis is more likely to be related to sepsis. Myoglobinuria is a feature of MH, but is a late sign. Suxamethonium is a recognised trigger for MH, but the fact of its use is not evidence for MH since the proportion of patients developing MH after suxamethonium is vanishingly small.

1. Association of Anaesthetists of Great Britain and Ireland guidelines for the management of a malignant hyperthermia (MH) crisis, 2011.
2. Larach MG, Gronert GA, Allen GC, *et al*. Clinical presentation, treatment, and complications of malignant hyperthermia in North America from 1987 to 2006. *Anaesth Analg* 2010; 110: 498-507.

 62 D

This patient has an unsurvivable brain injury. Your duty of care now rests with ensuring a dignified death commensurate with his wishes. In this situation, acting ethically in the 'best interests' of the patient can reasonably be interpreted as ensuring his wish to donate organs is carried out, and this allows for interventions such as central venous catheter placement and commencement of cardiovascular support to maximise the chances of a good outcome for the donated organs and their recipients. Guidance in the UK is provided by the NHS Blood and Transplant Service (NHSBT) and may vary in other countries.

Peripheral metaraminol is an option, but is not recommended as first line due to potential bradydysrhythmias. Expedition of the surgery in an untimely fashion is more likely to render a negative outcome for either the donor or recipients. Placement of a central line is recommended to gauge central venous pressure (CVP) and administer drugs, with low-dose vasopressin as the first-choice vasopressor. Brainstem death is associated with low vasopressin concentrations and as such this agent can be thought to restore 'normal physiological tone'. Noradrenaline can be utilised in addition as needed.

Whilst it is important to ensure normovolaemia, the avoidance of excessive fluid administration has been demonstrated to significantly increase the numbers of transplantable lungs in this cohort. An open access review article is available.

1. McKeown DW, Bonser RS, Kellum JA. Management of the heartbeating brain-dead organ donor *Br J Anaesth* 2012; 108(suppl 1): i96-i107.
2. Donor optimisation guideline for management of the brain-stem dead donor. http://www.odt.nhs.uk/donation/deceased-donation/donor-optimisation/resources/ (accessed 26th February 2015).

63 D

Synchronised DC shock should be administered to patients with a narrow complex tachycardia when adverse features are present. Adverse features include: shock, syncope, myocardial ischaemia and heart failure.

1. Resuscitation Council (UK). Resuscitation guidelines 2010. London, UK: Resuscitation Council (UK). http://www.resus.org.uk/pages/guide.htm (accessed 25th February 2015).

64 E

All options are plausible. However, the most likely diagnosis is E. Aortic myocardial infarction typically presents as a central crushing pain with autonomic features such as sweatiness and pallor. Rupture of a mitral valve may present as a decompensated heart failure picture. Boerhaave's syndrome is a spontaneous rupture of the oesophagus which may present as a sharp central chest pain radiating through to the back but has a time association with over-indulgence or repeated vomiting to raise intrathoracic pressure. A Type 1 myocardial infarction (i.e. due to plaque rupture or other non-interventional cause of acute coronary artery obstruction) could present as stated, but the cues suggest E is a better answer.

1. Miesel JL, Cottrell D. Differential diagnoses of chest pain in adults. www.uptodate.com/contents/differential-diagnosis-of-chest-pain-in-adult (accessed 24th July 2014).
2. Thygesen K, Alpert JS, Jaffe AS, *et al*. Third universal definition of myocardial infarction. *J Am Coll Cardiol* 2012; 60(16): 1581-98.

65 A

A retro-orbital haematoma with proptosis is a sight-threatening condition. Awake patients will often complain of extreme pain, ophthalmoplegia and visual disturbance. In sedated patients, clinical symptoms are negated and so extreme vigilance must be maintained. Retro-orbital pressure exerted on the optic nerve can cause rapid irreversible damage. Prompt recognition and action are vital.

A lateral canthotomy is the procedure of choice to decompress the orbit and release tension from the nerve. Although this is often performed by specialists, access to services may be restricted in certain circumstances. As a relatively simple sight-saving procedure, it should be understood by all those managing major trauma patients.

Neurosurgical decompression will do little to relieve retro-orbital pressure from local bleeding. Sonographic evaluation may reveal a swollen optic nerve sheath but this could be secondary to either local oedema following stretch or raised intracranial pressure (ICP). Hyperventilation may reduce ICP but this will not address the urgent issue. A Honan balloon can be used following the placement of a retrobulbar nerve block prior to ophthalmic surgery to reduce intra-ocular pressure through ocular massage, but is contraindicated in this situation.

A review article is available.

1.   McClenaghan FC, Ezra DG, Holmes SB. Mechanisms and management of vision loss following orbital and facial trauma. *Curr Opin Ophthalmol* 2011; 22(5): 426-31.

66 D

The patient's signs and symptoms are consistent with a diagnosis of meningitis or encephalitis. A raised protein level, a glucose <60% of plasma glucose and a pleocytosis of mainly mononuclear cells are strongly suggestive of TB meningitis. However it is worth noting that a polymorphonuclear or mixed pleocytosis does not exclude a diagnosis of

TB meningitis. India ink stain allows visualisation and diagnosis of *Cryptococcus*. Patients with HIV have an increased risk of cryptococcal meningitis and toxoplasmosis encephalitis but due to their immunosuppressed state they are more susceptible to all infections.

1.   Waldmann C, Soni N, Rhodes A. *Oxford Desk Reference Critical Care*. Oxford, UK: Oxford University Press, 2008.

67 A

The signs and symptoms of sepsis in pregnant women may be less distinctive than in the non-pregnant population and are not necessarily present in all cases; therefore, a high index of suspicion is necessary. All healthcare professionals should be aware of the symptoms and signs of maternal sepsis and critical illness, and of the rapid, potentially lethal course of severe sepsis and septic shock. Clinical signs of sepsis include one or more of the following: pyrexia, hypothermia, tachycardia, tachypnoea, hypoxia, hypotension, oliguria, impaired consciousness and failure to respond to treatment. These signs, including pyrexia, may not always be present and are not necessarily related to the severity of sepsis.

Regular observations of all vital signs (including temperature, pulse rate, blood pressure and respiratory rate) should be recorded on a Modified Early Obstetric Warning Score (MEOWS) chart or similar. A MEOWS chart should be used for all maternity inpatients to identify seriously ill pregnant women and refer them to critical care and obstetric anaesthetic colleagues according to local guidelines.

Early, goal-directed resuscitation has been shown to improve survival for non-pregnant patients presenting with septic shock. The Surviving Sepsis Campaign Resuscitation Bundle recommends that this is commenced pending transfer to an intensive care unit. The decision to transfer to intensive care should be decided by the critical care team in conjunction with the obstetric consultant and the consultant obstetric anaesthetist (levels III and IV evidence).

1.   Bacterial sepsis in pregnancy. Green-top guideline No. 64a. NHS Evidence, April 2012.

68   A

This patient is likely to have rhabdomyolysis with associated acute kidney injury and is developing severe hyperkalaemia and metabolic acidosis as a consequence. His clinical picture is one of progressive deterioration. As such his management must be aggressive. Oliguria for >12 hours is a listed indication for consideration of renal replacement therapy. Other indications include rapidly rising serum potassium, refractory acidosis, fluid overload and anuria. Given the magnitude of the insult, the rise in potassium and the fact that the patient has already had generous fluid resuscitation, renal replacement therapy would seem the most sensible option.

Alkalinisation of the urine appears to be losing support as a therapy, given the paucity of evidence. Increasing solubility of the Tamm-Horsfall urinary protein provides some face validity, but this must be balanced with the risks of hypocalcaemia following excess bicarbonate delivery. Having received 5L of intravenous fluid with minimal urinary response, there is little ground to suggest that this patient is not adequately fluid loaded. Further trials should be initiated, but titrated to fluid responsiveness rather than CVP measurement. Noradrenaline may well be needed to counteract the systemic inflammatory response, but there is no evidence to support supranormal goals. Initiation of insulin and dextrose is a reasonable temporizing measure to manage hyperkalaemia, but is unlikely to be sufficient given the clinical picture.

Induced diuresis with mannitol has some support, and may help remove circulating nephrotoxins through an osmotic diuretic effect. However, there are no RCT data to support its use and it is unlikely to constitute definitive care in this situation.

1.   Bosch X, Poch E, Grau JM. Current concepts. Rhabdomyolysis and acute kidney injury. *New Engl J Med* 2009; 361: 62-72.

69 B

Patients with rhabdomyolysis usually present with pigmented granular casts. Myoglobinuria causes a false-positive result for blood on urine dipstick as it is unable to distinguish between myoglobin and haemoglobin. Muscle breakdown releases intracellular contents including creatine kinase (CK) and phosphate, leading to raised CK and hyperphosphataemia. Hypocalcaemia results from calcium entering the damaged cells and from precipitation as calcium phosphate in necrotic tissue. In the later phases of rhabdomyolysis as renal function recovers, this calcium is mobilised and hypercalcaemia can result.

1.   Bosch X, Poch E, Grau JM. Current concepts. Rhabdomyolysis and acute kidney injury. *New Engl J Med* 2009; 361: 62-72.

70 C

Initial treatment will depend on the degree of hypercalcaemia and whether the patient is symptomatic from hypercalcaemia. In all cases, the patient's medications should be reviewed and contributing drugs (e.g. thiazide diuretics, calcium and vitamin D supplements) withheld.

Initial management is fluid rehydration. Patients who are asymptomatic with mild hypercalcaemia (serum calcium 2.6-2.9mmol/L) can usually be managed by encouraging oral fluid intake. Patients asymptomatic with moderate hypercalcaemia (serum calcium 3.0-3.4mmol/L) should receive intravenous fluid rehydration with 0.9% sodium chloride (typically 3-4L over the first 24 hours). Patients who are symptomatic with moderate hypercalcaemia (serum calcium 3.0-3.4mmol/L) or those with severe hypercalcaemia (serum calcium >3.4mmol/L) should receive vigorous rehydration using 0.9% sodium chloride to restore extracellular volume (patients frequently require 3-6L over the first 24 hours). This requires careful monitoring to avoid complications of fluid overload.

Paper 3 Answers

Intravenous bisphosphonates are the treatment of choice in volume-replete individuals where hypercalcaemia persists despite rehydration and the parathyroid hormone (PTH) level is suppressed. When volume-replete, patients should have serum calcium rechecked (typically after 24 hours). Patients with persistent serum hypercalcaemia >3.0mmol/L and suppressed PTH should receive an intravenous bisphosphonate. Patients with hypercalcaemia due to a high concentration of parathyroid hormone-related peptide (PTHrP — a protein produced by some tumours) have a poorer response to bisphosphonate therapy.

A biochemical response is usually seen within 2-4 days of treatment and the lowest serum calcium level seen at 7-10 days. Although there is a temptation to repeat bloods straight away, it is advisable to routinely remeasure serum calcium after 5-7 days after definitive treatment with bisphosphonate.

The use of intravenous furosemide should be reserved for patients with features of volume overload following fluid rehydration. Occasionally, haemodialysis may be required, supervised by a renal physician with adjustment of the concentration of calcium in diasylate.

1. Walji N, Chan AK, Peake DR. Common acute oncological emergencies: diagnosis, investigation and management. *Postgrad Med J* 2008; 84: 418-27.

71 A

Pain is a serious issue for the practising intensivist and a routine part of day-to-day practice. Whilst opiate analgaesia provides the mainstay of care, it is important to recognise the potential benefits of adjuvant strategies. A summary review has been recently published. Ketamine in subanaesthetic dosage provides a useful rescue and potential adjuvant strategy for patients with challenging pain issues. A Cochrane review has previously highlighted use and confirmed the benefits, including a reduction in opioid consumption and a decrease in the incidence of nausea and vomiting at 24 hours.

Pregabalin as a preventative strategy has shown some promise in the reduction of chronic post-surgical pain. Optimum use is pre-operative, the onset of effect is not immediate and some surgeons have raised concerns regarding the administration of enteric medications through feeding gastrostomy/jejunostomy tubing early in the course of recovery. Intra-operative lidocaine can decrease opiate consumption, but has a limited role in the awake postoperative patient. Clonidine is currently under investigation as an adjuvant analgaesic, but has little role for the patient who is already hypotensive and on α-stimulation. NSAIDs are relatively contraindicated in a patient with peptic ulcer disease and precarious renal function following major surgery.

1.   Ramaswamy S, Wilson JA, Colvin L. Non-opioid-based adjuvant analgaesia in perioperative care. *Contin Educ Anaesth Crit Care Pain* 2013; 13(5): 152-7.
2.   Bell RF, Dahl JB, Moore RA, Kalso EA. Perioperative ketamine for acute postoperative pain. *Cochrane Database Syst Rev* 2006; 1: CD004603.
3.   Bonin RP, Orser BA, Englesakis M, *et al*. The prevention of chronic postsurgical pain using gabapentin and pregabalin: a combined systematic review and meta-analysis. *Anesth Analg* 2012; 115: 428-42
4.   http://clinicaltrials.gov/show/NCT01082874 (accessed 26th February 2015).

 72   D

Botulism is caused by an exotoxin released from *Clostridium botulinum*. It is characterised by a descending motor paralysis affecting primarily cranial, respiratory and autonomic nerves. Tetanus causes skeletal muscle ridigity and spasm. Syringobulbia is the development of fluid cavities within the brainstem, which may interrupt motor, sensory and autonomic nerve pathways. Presentation is usually with a gradual worsening of symptoms and the lack of sensory features is against the diagnosis in this case. In Guillain-Barré syndrome, an ascending and symmetrical weakness is seen, with sensory and autonomic disturbances. Myasthenia gravis has a relapsing, remitting course and while it may present with diplopia and dysphagia, symmetrical weakness is unlikely and there is no autonomic involvement.

1.   Waldmann C, Soni N, Rhodes A. *Oxford Desk Reference Critical Care.* Oxford, UK: Oxford University Press, 2008.

73 E

This man is clearly septic with evidence of septic shock. His volume status has been improved by intravenous crystalloid therapy at a rate recommended by the Surviving Sepsis Campaign (SSC) guidance but he is now demonstrating signs of fluid repletion with a CVP of 12mmHg (the utility of CVP as a marker of volume status is a subject for debate but is still a SSC recommendation). The next most appropriate step is now intravenous vasopressor therapy, and norepinephrine is most appropriate via central venous access. Following initial resuscitative measures, sepsis resuscitation algorithms advocate the use of blood transfusion and inotropic support to improve oxygen delivery to the tissues if markers of tissue perfusion and oxygen extraction (lactate and $ScvO_2$) remain deranged.

1.   Surviving Sepsis Campaign. International guidelines for management of severe sepsis and septic shock, 2012. http://www.sccm.org/Documents/SSC-Guidelines.pdf (accessed 20th September 2014).

74 E

Clearing the C-spine in the obtunded trauma patient has presented a dilemma to intensivists, radiologists, neurosurgeons and spinal surgeons for many years. The theoretical risk of an unstable ligamentous injury undetected by CT has left many clinicians feeling reluctant to discontinue spinal precautions until definitive soft tissue imaging is obtained.

There is little evidence to support this approach and it is not without risk. Spinal precautions have no supporting evidence to suggest benefit at recent systematic review and can cause complications such as airway obstruction, local ulceration and more importantly in this case, obstruction of venous drainage and a raised ICP. In addition, multiple series have been published assessing the incidence of missed spinal injury detected on MR imaging requiring surgical intervention in this patient cohort, with rates usually <1%.

In this case it would seem prudent to focus on ICP management and discontinue all precautions, especially in the presence of a consultant reported CT scan. Nursing in the midline ensures a limited range of cervical rotation/lateral flexion until the case can be reviewed by the multidisciplinary team. If clinical concerns of spinal injury continue to exist, then MR imaging is the gold standard. There is little to be achieved by continued immobilisation in a sedated and ventilated patient during this phase.

1. Kwan I, Bunn F, Roberts IG. Spinal immobilisation for trauma patients. *Cochrane Database Syst Rev* 2001; 2: CD002803.
2. Hogan GJ, Mirvis SE, Shanmuganathan K, Scalea TM. Exclusion of unstable cervical spine injury in obtunded patients with blunt trauma: is MR imaging needed when multi-detector row CT findings are normal? *Radiology* 2005; 237(1): 106-13.

75 A

The combination of symptoms seen in this patient is highly suggestive of thyroid storm. Pyrexia is not generally a feature of decompensated alcoholic liver disease and sepsis is unlikely given the normal white cell count and inflammatory markers. Patients with malaria usually present with fever, headache and malaise, and gastrointestinal, jaundice and respiratory symptoms can be seen; however, tachyarrhythmias and cardiac failure are not normally present. Thyroid storm represents the extreme in the spectrum of thyrotoxicosis where decompensation of organ function can occur. The transition into the state of thyroid storm usually requires a second superimposed insult: most commonly infection, although trauma, surgery, myocardial infarction, diabetic ketoacidosis, pregnancy and parturition can also precipitate the condition. Any of the classical signs and symptoms of the thyrotoxic state may be seen. Pyrexia is almost universal (>39°C) and when present in an unwell patient with known thyrotoxicosis, should prompt immediate consideration of thyroid storm.

Cardiac decompensation (usually due to high-output failure), tachyarrhythmias (usually atrial in origin), neurological dysfunction (agitation, delirium or psychosis), liver dysfunction (secondary to cardiac failure,

Paper 3 Answers

hypoperfusion or a direct effect of excess thyroid hormone), nausea and vomiting, abdominal pain and jaundice are all features seen in cases of thyroid storm. The diagnosis of thyroid storm must be made on the basis of suspicious but non-specific clinical findings. Treatment includes supportive measures and thyroid-specific therapies to block synthesis, block release, block T4 to T3 conversion and block enterohepatic circulation.

1.   Lalloo DG, Shingadia D, Pasvol G, et al. UK malaria treatment guidelines. J Infect 2007; 54: 111-21.
2.   Carroll R, Matfin G. Endocrine and metabolic emergencies: thyroid storm. Ther Adv Endocrinol Metab 2010; 1(3): 139-45.

76 E

This case suggests atrial fibrillation with rapid ventricular response with haemodynamic instability. As per the Advanced Life Support guidance, this patient has adverse features (chest pain and signs of shock) and requires urgent DC cardioversion. Carotid sinus massage has a role in the management of regular narrow complex tachycardia, but not fast atrial fibrillation.

1.   Resuscitation Council (UK). Advanced life support 2011. London, UK: Resuscitation Council (UK). https://www.resus.org.uk/pages/als.pdf (accessed 25th February 2015).

77 A

Stroke remains a huge healthcare burden with a distinct impact on intensive care workload. An understanding of the classification symptoms, urgent management and prognosis are vital for practising intensivists, in order to facilitate appropriate emergency care and recognise futility.

The advent of thrombolysis and early treatments for stroke has been hampered by problems identifying those in need. As such, NICE guidance endorses both the pre-hospital FAST (Face, Arm, Speech, Time to call 999) recognition test and the emergency department ROSIER (Recognition of Stroke in the Emergency Room) scoring systems to streamline decision making in urgent stroke care. The ROSIER score is reduced if fits or loss of consciousness are present, and increased if visual field defects, asymmetric weakness or dysphasia are present. A ROSIER score of >0 is strongly suggestive of cerebrovascular accident with a sensitivity of 92%. All the component parts are available within the case description to calculate this score, which would be 3.

Classification of stroke syndromes allows the early prognosis and directed care. The Bamford classification is the commonest in use at present. A diagnosis of total anterior circulation infarct (TACS) is made when all of homonymous hemianopia, higher cerebral dysfunction and unilateral hemiparesis are present; whereas a partial anterior circulation infarct (PACS) requires only two of the three. The high 30-day mortality of a TACS (40%) is reduced ten-fold with a PACS.

Emergent intubation compromises the ongoing clinical assessment regarding neurological signs, and as such should be carefully considered rather than mandated. There is no overt suggestion of airway danger in this scenario and it may well be possible to obtain imaging with a dedicated escort only. Thrombolysis carries a large remit of supporting evidence up to a cut-off of 4.5 hours and as such is recommended by NICE, although concerns persist and the debate continues. The recent IST-3 (International Stroke Trial) study notably demonstrated no difference between patients thrombolysed or not between 4.5-6 hours and as such cannot be used to support extended thrombolysis periods. NICE guidance recommends antiplatelet agents for newly diagnosed atrial fibrillation for up to 14 days prior to initiating therapeutic anticoagulation, in order to avoid haemorrhagic transformation of the infarct.

1. Raithatha A, Pratt G, Rash A. Developments in the management of acute ischaemic stroke: implications for anaesthetic and critical care management. *Contin Educ Anaesth Crit Care Pain* 2013; 13(3): 80-6
2. The National Institute for Health and Care Excellence. Stroke: diagnosis and initial management of acute stroke and transient ischaemic attack (TIA). NICE clinical guideline 68. London, UK: NICE, 2008. www.nice.org.uk (accessed 25th February 2015).
3. Nor AM, Davis J, Sen B, *et al*. The Recognition of Stroke in the Emergency Room (ROSIER) Scale: development and validation of a stroke recognition instrument. *Lancet Neurol* 2005; 4(11): 727-34.
4. The IST3 Collaborators group. The benefits and harms of intravenous thrombolysis with recombinant tissue plasminogen activator within 6h of acute ischaemic stroke (the third international stroke trial [IST-3]): a randomised controlled trial. *Lancet* 2012; 379(9834): 2352-63.

Paper 3 Answers

78 B

NICE guidelines state that non-invasive ventilation (NIV) should be considered for all COPD patients with a persisting respiratory acidosis after 1 hour of standard medical therapy. Standard medical therapy should include controlled oxygen to maintain SaO_2 88-92%, nebulised salbutamol, nebulised ipratropium, prednisolone and an antibiotic if indicated. Patients with a pH <7.26 may benefit from NIV but they have a higher risk of treatment failure and should be managed in a high dependency or ICU setting. As this patient has a persisting respiratory acidosis with a pH of 7.24 after an hour of optimal management, he should be transferred to a critical care area for a trial of NIV. A management plan should be put in place should he fail to improve with this therapy. There is currently minimal evidence for the use of aminophylline in the management of an exacerbation of COPD. This, along with its high incidence of side effects, means that it is only recommended in cases where all other management has failed. Ketamine has a role in intractable asthma but is not used in the management of exacerbations of COPD. The evidence base supporting the use of doxapram is very limited.

1.   British Thoracic Society, Royal College of Physicians, The Intensive Care Society. The use of non-invasive ventilation in the management of patients with COPD admitted to hospital with acute type II respiratory failure (with particular reference to bilevel positive pressure ventilation). London, UK: RCP, 2008.
2.   Town GI. Aminophylline for COPD exacerbations? Not usually. *Thorax* 2005; 60: 709.

79 C

The clinical history suggests the possibility of tricyclic antidepressant poisoning. Toxicity is mainly due to anticholinergic (atropine-like) effects at autonomic nerve endings and in the brain. The most important electrocardiographic (ECG) feature of toxicity is prolongation of the QRS interval, which indicates a high risk of progression to ventricular tachycardia. In this case, given that the ventricular rate is 130bpm, this is likely to be a sinus tachycardia with prolonged QRS duration rather than a ventricular tachycardia which would usually have a much higher rate.

Tachyarrhythmias are most appropriately treated by correction of hypoxia and acidosis. Even in the absence of acidosis, 50mmol of sodium bicarbonate should be given by intravenous infusion to adults with arrhythmias or clinically significant QRS prolongation on the ECG. Alkalinisation promotes dissociation of the tricyclic antidepressant molecule from cardiac sodium channels and therefore reduces cardiotoxicity. There are reports of phenytoin use in the treatment of tricyclic poisoning, but it is not first-line and should only be used under specialist instruction due to the potential for worsening arrhythmias. Intravenous benzodiazepines may be needed if repeated seizures occur.

1.   MHRA. Amitriptyline overdose. http://www.mhra.gov.uk (accessed 14th July 2014).
2.   Foianini A, Joseph Wiegand T, Benowitz N. What is the role of lidocaine or phenytoin in tricyclic antidepressant-induced cardiotoxicity? *Clin Toxicol* 2010; 48(4): 325-30.
3.   Hoffman JR, Votey SR, Bayer M, Silver L. Effect of hypertonic sodium bicarbonate in the treatment of moderate-to-severe cyclic antidepressant overdose. *Am J Emerg Med* 1993; 11: 336-41.

80   E

Management of the post-cardiac arrest syndrome continues to develop. Although attention must be paid to the potential causes of arrest and identification of the underlying pathology, the syndrome in itself requires treatment in order to optimise outcome. The balance between these two interests can sometimes be conflicting.

The recent literature would suggest that 36°C is equally efficacious to 33°C with regard to post-arrest management. As such, the institution of further cooling at a temperature of 35.6°C will likely achieve little benefit, although pyrexia should be aggressively managed. Loading with antiplatelet therapy confers significant bleeding risk in this age group. At present there is no hard evidence of acute Type 1 myocardial infarction. The possibility of non-ST elevation myocardial infarction remains. The recent ACCOAST (A Comparison of Prasugrel at the Time of Percutaneous Coronary Intervention or as Pre-treatment At the Time of Diagnosis in Patients with Non-ST-Elevation Myocardial Infarction) trial supports conservative management of such cases prior to definitive percutaneous coronary intervention. Bronchoscopy is not indicated to improve gas exchange and is unlikely to help in the acute setting. A CT brain may be indicated to exclude additional pathology (although the history given is suggestive of a primary coronary cause of cardiac arrest), but plays little role in early prognostication of an elderly patient with such a short downtime.

Hyperoxia has been recently suggested to adversely influence outcome post-cardiac arrest in large cohort studies. It is a rapid simple measure to influence and may have significant impact on morbidity and mortality. As such, titrating down FiO_2 is the most suitable immediate intervention of the above options.

1. Nielsen N, Wetterslev I, Cronberg T, *et al*. Targeted temperature management at 33°C versus 36°C after cardiac arrest. *N Engl J Med* 2013; 369: 2197-206.
2. Montalescot G, Bolognese L, Dudek D, *et al*. Pretreatment with prasugrel in non-ST-segment elevation acute coronary syndromes. *N Engl J Med* 2013; 369: 999-1010.
3. Kilgannon JH, Jones AE, Shapiro N, *et al*. Association between arterial hyperoxia following resuscitation from cardiac arrest and in-hospital mortality *JAMA* 2010; 303(21): 2165-71.

81 D

This patient is clearly compromised by her bradycardia and immediate action must be undertaken to increase her heart rate. If there is no electrical output at the pacing wire tips when the set pacing mode calls for such an output, this is termed 'failure to pace'. This can be due to lead malfunction or unstable connections, insufficient power (necessitating a battery change), cross-talk inhibition and oversensing. 'Failure to capture' is when there is electrical output at the pacemaker wire tips (confirmed by visible pacing spikes on the ECG), but this does not cause a cardiac contraction, as shown by the absence of a mechanical cardiac impulse on the arterial pressure or pulse oximeter waveform. The cause is an increase in the resistance at the wire/myocardium interface, most commonly due to fibrosis around the pacemaker lead.

Failure to capture is the commonest problem encountered with temporary epicardial pacing. If the capture threshold has increased, increasing the output from the pacemaker should cause mechanical capture and rectify the problem. If the threshold is progressively increasing and the patient is dependent on the pacemaker, an alternative means of stimulus delivery should be put in place before capture is entirely lost.

1. Reade MC. Temporary epicardial pacing after cardiac surgery: a practical review. Part 2: Selection of epicardial pacing modes and troubleshooting. *Anaesthesia* 2007; 62: 364-73.

82 C

Pneumocystis jiroveci pneumonia (PJP) is a serious complication of anti-rejection therapy used in solid organ transplant patients. The incidence in moderately immunosuppressed renal transplant recipients is low (around 0.6%), and therefore co-trimoxazole prophylaxis is not routinely given. However, episodes of rejection may require treatment with high-dose methylprednisolone, anti-thymocyte globulin and other agents which greatly increase the risk. Given the clinical history of significant hypoxia, recent immunosuppression (implied) and unremarkable chest X-ray, PJP is a likely diagnosis and of the options given only bronchoalveolar lavage is likely to provide diagnostic information.

1. MacCaughan JA, Courtney AE *Pneumocystis jiroveci* pneumonia in renal transplantation: time to review our practice? *Nephrol Dial Transplant* 2012; 27(1): 13-5.

83 B

This is a likely presentation of staphylococcal toxic shock syndrome, an acute toxin-mediated multi-system disorder with a high morbidity and mortality. Presentation features can be very subtle. Previous associations with retained tampon use are no longer directly applicable following manufacture changes and advice leaflets resulting in a reduction of incidence to 1/100,000 in the USA. It must be considered with any condition where underlying *Staphylococcus* infection is suspected. In particular, pain out of proportion to that expected can herald an underlying infectious myositis. Systemic upset is also a suggestive symptom.

Early aggressive antimicrobial treatment and source control are the mainstay of therapy. Antimicrobial therapy has a dual rationale — bacteriocidal antibiotics are indicated to prevent spreading infection but bacteriostatic antibiotics can result in decreased toxin production and thus limit the associated multi-organ morbidity. To this end, standard bacteriocidal therapy is often combined with either clindamycin or linezolid, with the latter having the sole aim of 'switching off' toxin production. Penicillins are recommended with the addition of vancomycin or linezolid in cases of suspected *Streptococcus pyogenes*, although all antibiotic decisions should be guided by local expert advice.

Intravenous immunoglobulin has a potential role, but limited supporting evidence. It is recommended for progressive disease despite adequate source control and antimicrobial therapy. Although this is a true surgical emergency and extensive debridement may well be necessary, time to antimicrobial therapy is a critical determinant of survival in these cases and as such should be paramount. A recent review article is available covering these discussion points.

1. Lappin E, Ferguson AJ. Gram-positive toxic shock syndromes. *Lancet Infect Dis* 2009; 9: 281-90.

84   E

The most likely underlying problem is abdominal compartment syndrome (ACS). Medical management of raised intra-abdominal pressure should be instigated. The World Society of the Abdominal Compartment Syndrome (WSACS) defines intra-abdominal pressure (IAP) as the steady-state pressure concealed within the abdominal cavity. In critically ill adults, IAP is approximately 5-7mmHg. Intra-abdominal hypertension (IAH) is defined as a sustained or repeated pathological elevation in IAP of 12 or more mmHg. Abdominal compartment syndrome is defined as a sustained IAP >20mmHg (with or without an abdominal perfusion pressure [APP] <60mmHg) that is associated with new organ dysfunction/failure. Grade I IAH has an IAP 12-15mmHg, Grade II 16-20mmHg, Grade III 21-25mmHg and Grade IV >25mmHg. Risk factors for IAH and ACS include:

factors which decrease abdominal wall compliance, increase intraluminal contents, increase intra-abdominal contents and cause capillary leak/fluid resuscitation. Other risk factors include age, mechanical ventilation, positive end-expiratory pressure (PEEP) >10cmH$_2$O, obesity, peritonitis, sepsis and hypotension. If a patient's IAP is consistently greater than 11mmHg, medical management should be instigated to reduce IAP. These measures include evacuation of intraluminal contents, evacuation of intra-abdominal space-occupying lesions, improving abdominal wall compliance, optimising fluid administration and optimising systemic/regional perfusion. This patient does not meet the criteria for renal replacement therapy for acute kidney injury. While renal replacement therapy with fluid removal may be used to decrease intra-abdominal pressure, this is not currently recommended by the WSACS. Excessive fluid resuscitation should be avoided as this can worsen IAP. Due to the recent surgery, prokinetics and laxatives should not be administered. Increasing his sedation and analgesia will improve abdominal wall compliance and, therefore, hopefully, reduce IAP and improve renal perfusion. Should this fail to improve his IAP, further medical measures should be instigated and if these fail, decompressive laparotomy should be considered.

1.   Kirkpatrick AW, Roberts DJ, De Waele J, et al. Intra-abdominal hypertension and the abdominal compartment syndrome: updated consensus definitions and clinical practice guidelines from the World Society of the Abdominal Compartment Syndrome. *Intensive Care Med* 2013; 39: 1190-206.
2.   Hall NA, Fox AJ. Renal replacement therapies in critical care. *Contin Educ Anaesth Crit Care Pain* 2006; 6(5): 197-202.

85   E

The fluid resuscitation aims to restore tissue perfusion, avoiding end-organ ischaemia, preserving viable tissue and minimising tissue oedema. The Parkland formula is a guide and fluid resuscitation should be titrated against clinical response, invasive monitoring and urine output (0.5ml/kg/hr).

Invasive monitoring is necessary in the severely burnt patient to help guide both volume replacement and the use of inotropes. The term 'fluid creep' describes the excessive volumes of fluid used for resuscitation which has occurred in some burn patients with complications. Hypokalaemia, hypophosphataemia, hypocalcaemia, and hypomagnesaemia are common and should be treated. There is a phenomenon known as 'burn shock' which describes a combination of hypovolaemic, distributive, and cardiogenic shock which is refractory to massive intravenous resuscitation.

Of the choices given, central venous pressure and mean arterial pressure are both poor markers of adequacy of fluid resuscitation even in non-burns patients, and heart rate will be rapid due to a variety of factors including pain and the severe inflammatory response. Urine output is a surrogate of end-organ perfusion, and is likely to be the most useful initial marker of the adequacy of organ perfusion, with the caveat that acute kidney injury is likely to develop secondary to critical illness and rhabdomyolysis over time, and renal biochemistry should be closely monitored.

1.   Bishop S, Maguire S. Anaesthesia and intensive care for major burns. *Contin Educ Anaesth Crit Care Pain* 2012; 12(3): 118-22.

86 D

This patient unfortunately appears to have multiple organ failure — neurological, hepatological, cardiovascular and renal. Prognosis in this situation, especially in the absence of a reversible precipitant would be very bleak. Recent data would suggest that following three-organ failure, mortality approaches 90-100%.

Interestingly enough, generic organ failure scores appear to perform better at predicting outcome than specific liver disease scoring systems. At recent systematic review, the SOFA score performed best with an area under the receiver operating characteristic curve (AUC) of >0.9, reporting excellent discrimination. In contrast, the Child-Pugh score demonstrated an AUC of 0.6-0.7 and the MELD score noted an AUC of approximately 0.8. As such, if you were seeking to discriminate likely survival, the SOFA score would be the best choice to guide clinical decision making in an acute situation.

The APACHE II score also performs reasonably well. The Glasgow Alcohol Score is a tool designed to predict the need for steroid therapy in acute alcoholic hepatitis.

1. Flood S, Bodenham A, Jackson P. Mortality of patients with alcoholic liver disease admitted to critical care: a systematic review. *J Intensive Care Soc* 2012; 13(2): 130-5.

87 B

To differentiate between causes of weakness, electrophysiological investigations are used. Motor response is elicited by supramaximal electrical stimulation of an extremity nerve, with recording from an appropriate distal muscle innervated by that nerve. The compound muscle action potential (CMAP) is the summated response of all stimulated muscle fibres within that muscle. Stimulation at two points along the nerve is required to calculate motor nerve conduction velocity. Sensory (or mixed) nerve action potential (SNAP) is obtained by supramaximal stimulation of a sensory or mixed nerve, with recording electrodes placed along the same nerve. Distal motor and sensory latencies, motor and sensory conduction velocity, amplitude of CMAP and SNAP, and waveforms of these potentials are noted. Abnormality of conduction strongly favours a neuropathic process. In axonal neuropathy, CMAP and SNAP amplitude are reduced (e.g. critical illness polyneuropathy). Demyelinating neuropathy is characterised by slowing of conduction (e.g. Guillain-Barré syndrome). Repetitive nerve stimulation uses a train of 10 supramaximal stimuli at 2-3Hz. A >10% decrement of CMAP amplitude from the first to the fourth response is significant and indicates compromise of neuromuscular transmission, as seen in myasthenia gravis. Pre-synaptic neuromuscular junction disorders, e.g. Lambert-Eaton syndrome and botulism, have low baseline CMAP amplitude. An increment response of >100% can be elicited following a 10-second exercise of muscle being tested or with fast (20-50Hz) repetitive stimulation. Patients with critical illness myopathy often have elevated blood creatine phosphokinase concentrations. Electrophysiological tests show reduced CMAP amplitude, normal SNAP amplitude and normal conduction velocities, and muscle necrosis is usually apparent on histology. Patients with critical illness polyneuropathy show a generalised, symmetrical, flaccid weakness with cranial nerve sparing, which usually presents in the recovery phase of a severe systemic illness. Electrophysiological features are consistent with axonal degeneration and show low amplitude of CMAP and SNAP, with near normal conduction velocity.

1.	Dhand UK. Clinical approach to the weak patient in the intensive care unit. *Respir Care* 2006; 51(9): 1024-41.
2.	Appleton R, Kinsella J. Intensive care unit-acquired weakness. *Contin Educ Anaesth Crit Care Pain* 2012; 12(2): 62-6.

88 E

According to the UK National Guidelines for HIV Testing 2008, the following are AIDS-defining illnesses based on systems:

* Respiratory — tuberculosis, pneumocystis.
* Neurological — cerebral toxoplasmosis, primary cerebral lymphoma, cryptococcal meningitis, progressive multifocal leucoencephalopathy.
* Dermatology — Kaposi's sarcoma.
* Gastroenterology — persistent cryptosporidiosis.
* Oncology — non-Hodgkin's lymphoma.
* Gynaecology — cervical cancer.
* Ophthamology — CMV retinitis.

Persistent oral candidiasis is not an AIDS-defining illness, but is one of a list of conditions that should prompt clinicians to consider HIV testing.

1.	British HIV Association (BHIVA). UK national guidelines for HIV testing, 2008. http://www.bhiva.org (accessed 20th July 2014).

89 E

This patient has been asleep during a house fire. As such, it is unlikely that the reason for her obtunded state will be traumatic in origin. A CT brain may be appropriate given the low GCS, but a whole body CT seems unwarranted. Far more likely is the presence of either carbon monoxide poisoning or moderate to severe cyanide poisoning.

Acute cyanide inhalation can present as a result of prolonged smoke exposure during a house fire, when certain substances including wool, silk, polyurethane and rubber are burnt. Symptoms of moderate poisoning include headache and dizziness proceeding to loss of consciousness, coma and fixed unreactive pupils. Arterial blood gas analysis will reveal a fixed metabolic acidosis with a high anion gap and a markedly raised lactate, secondary to cytotoxic hypoxia and anaerobic cellular respiration. A cyanide assay is available but performed in few departments. As such, patients with a suggestive history and clinical features in keeping with moderate to severe cyanide poisoning should receive empirical antidote therapy. Treatment options include sodium thiosulphate, dicobalt edetate and hydroxocobalamin.

Although carbon monoxide poisoning can present in a similar manner, treatment is principally through inhalation of high concentrations of oxygen, which is already occurring in this case. The evidence for hyperbaric therapy is equivocal, and it is no longer recommended by the National Poisons Information Service in the United Kingdom, regardless of the severity of toxicity. It is still recommended in many other countries, and is usually considered if levels are >40%, although patients may be treated with lower levels if cardiovascular or neurological impairment is present.

Whole body CT is unlikely to reveal any extensive injuries given the absence of mechanism and will cause a significant delay in treatment, although a CT brain would not be an unreasonable investigation to exclude an intracranial cause of the low GCS. Further fluid and inotropic support are warranted but will do little to definitively manage the underlying cause for the profound lactic acidosis.

1. http://lifeinthefastlane.com/cyanide-poisoning (accessed 26th February 2015).
2. Hammel J. A review of acute cyanide poisoning with a treatment update. *Crit Care Nurse* 2011; 31: 172-82.
3. http://www.toxbase.org/Poisons-Index-A-Z/C-Products/Carbon-monoxide-A (accessed 26th February 2015).

90 B

It is important to note that this situation needs experienced anaesthetic and surgical personnel, and different techniques may be preferred depending on the clinical circumstances and the experience of the clinicians involved. There is no single right answer, but B is given as such based on local expert opinion in the Editor's institution. The reference below illustrates that even experts disagree.

An ABC assessment shows that her airway is at risk. Releasing the sutures or clips can sometimes allow evacuation of the haematoma if it is superficial or a release of the pressure effects. In this case the patient remains with a rapidly deteriorating airway which should be secured at the earliest opportunity. As she has recently eaten, gas or intravenous induction or use of a laryngeal mask would put her at risk of aspiration and should therefore be avoided. However, the laryngeal mask should certainly be part of any back-up plan to maintain oxygenation in the event of an inability to intubate the trachea. Administration of atracurium would be hazardous and in the event of difficulty maintaining oxygenation, the patient would not recover the ability to breathe spontaneously for some time.

Of the remaining options, none is ideal. Awake tracheostomy under local anaesthetic would be safe if practical, but given that this patient is in extremis and thrashing around the bed, it is unlikely she would allow this to occur. Similarly, it seems unlikely that the patient would tolerate awake fibre-optic intubation, although this might be an option with the use of sedation in very experienced hands. Given the stridor and bleeding into the tissues around the airway, the airway anatomy is likely to be distorted and a rapid sequence induction could worsen the situation into a can't ventilate, can't intubate scenario. However, most airway experts would concur that this is the least worst option; if this is attempted it should be in theatre with a surgeon in attendance ready to gain access to the trachea in the event of difficulty intubating the trachea and/or ventilating the patient. Appropriate skilled assistance and a variety of difficult airway equipment should be immediately available.

1.   Cook TM1, Morgan PJ, Hersch PE. Equal and opposite expert opinion. Airway obstruction caused by a retrosternal thyroid mass: management and prospective international expert opinion. *Anaesthesia* 2011; 66(9): 828-36.